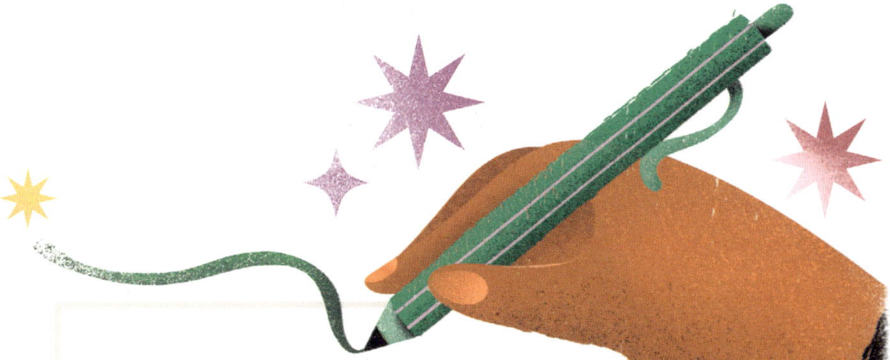

This journal belongs to:

Name ....

Email ....

Telephone ....

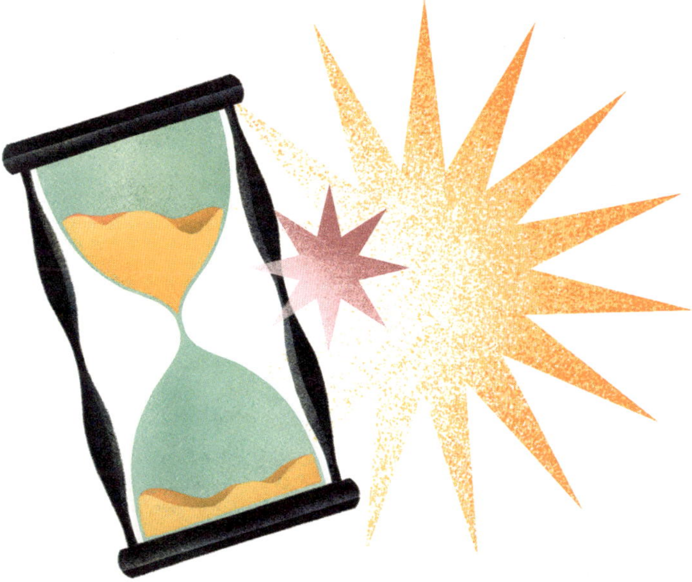

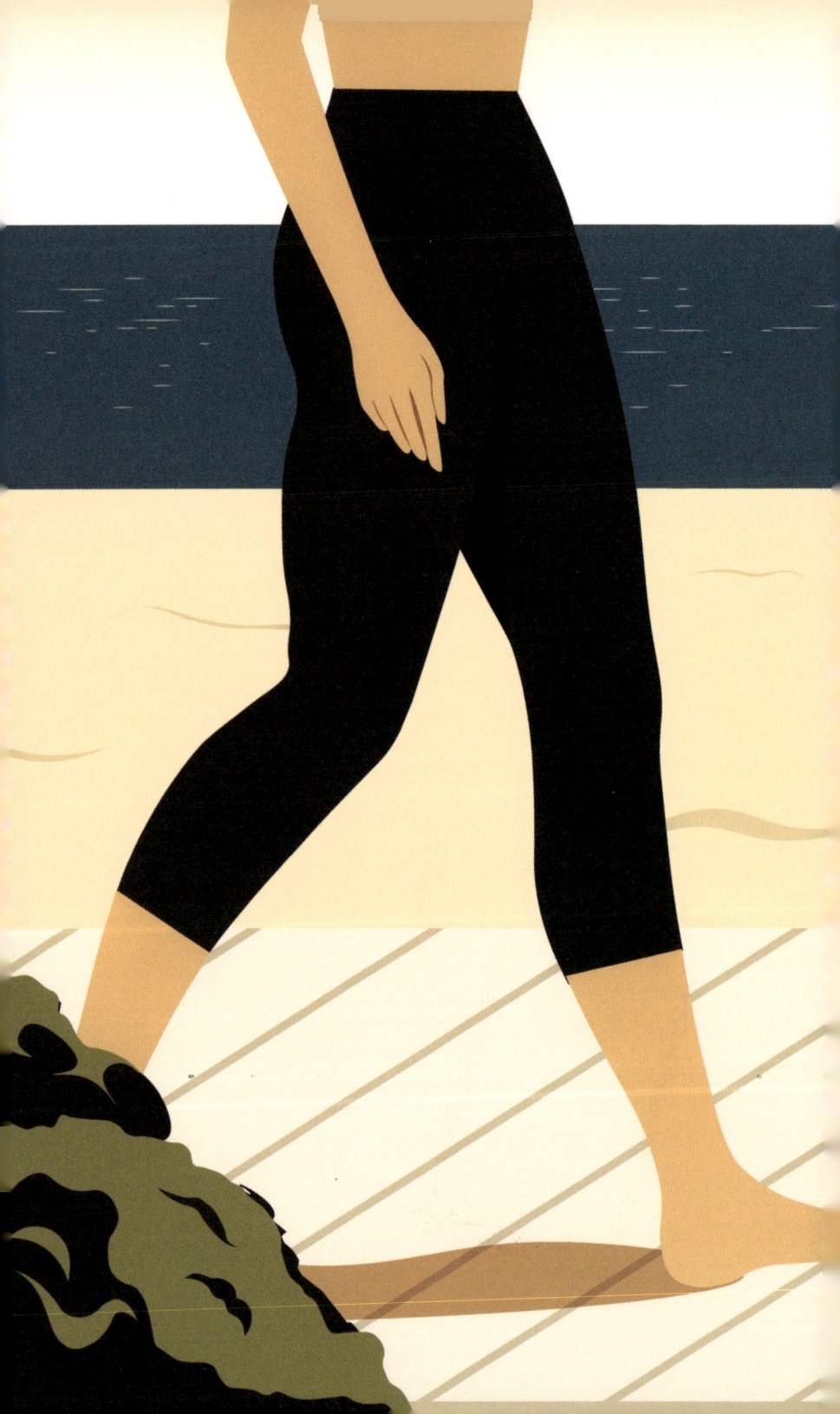

Breathe
Meditation
JOURNAL

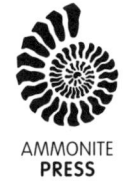

AMMONITE
PRESS

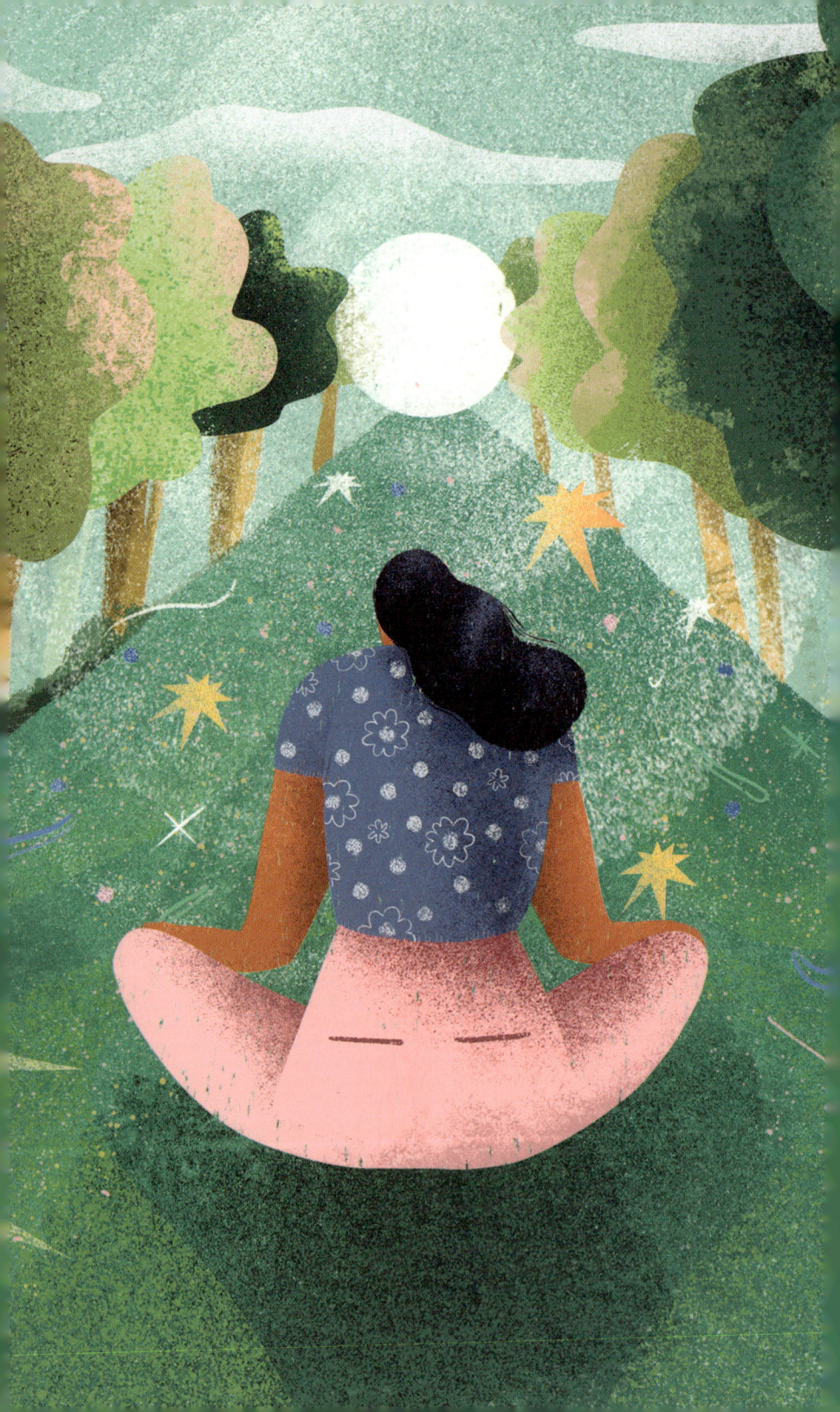

Meditation

In the past you might have added a daily meditation practice to a list of things you'd love to have time to get around to, in much the same way as learning another language or playing a musical instrument. But embracing meditation is about more than establishing a new hobby. Setting a few minutes aside each day for contemplation can be wholly transformative.

Opening up, allowing yourself to feel vulnerable, accepting whatever emotions arise – these are the fundamentals of meditation and the foundations for spiritual growth. Learn to slow racing thoughts, let go of negativity and become increasingly aware of where you're placing your attention. With no attachment to preconceived ideas of how things should be or should go, you are free to simply be as you are.

With its beautifully illustrated articles filled with science-based advice, mindful exercises and space to express thoughts and feelings, this journal is a doorway to exploring the type of meditation practice that works best for you. Use it to move from trying to influence and control your thoughts and emotions, to accepting and welcoming them, and discover a different way of living.

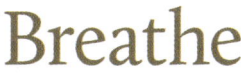

breathemagazine.com

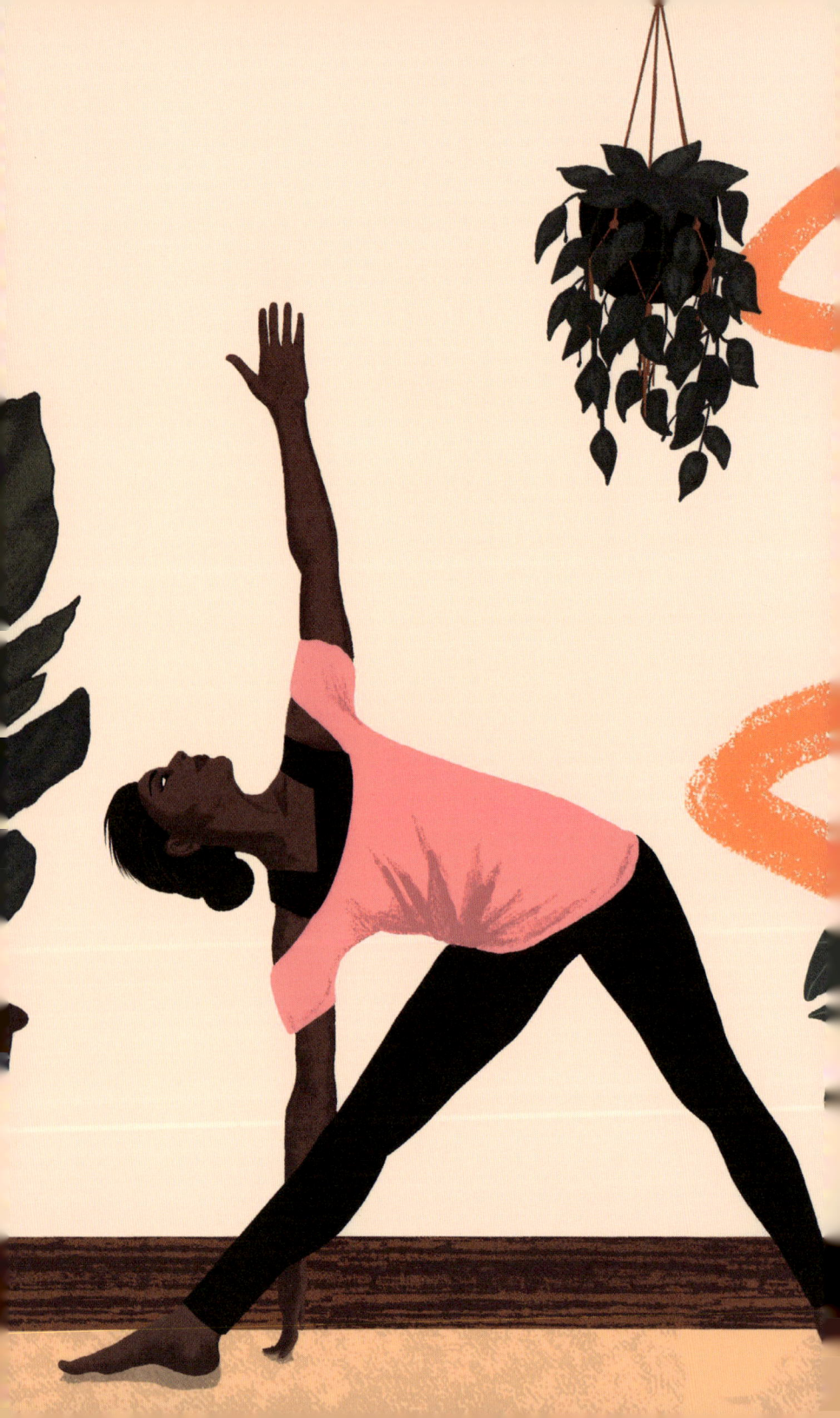

Contents

The long view 8

Ahead of the curve 16

Discomfort zone 24

DIY wellness weekend 32

Manifestly for you 40

Open invitation 48

Parts of the story 58

Behind the mask 68

Into the blue 78

Swerve from your path 84

It's not you, it's me 92

Cogs in motion 102

Reawaken the senses 110

Slowly but surely 120

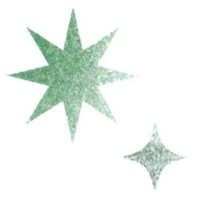

The long view

There are various ways to squeeze a short but powerful meditation session into the day and reap the benefits, but what are the advantages of extending it to an hour or more? A long-time practitioner guides us through

The idea of emulating the tradition of Buddhist monks and spending hours – if not days – meditating, might seem fanciful to many. After all, a lifestyle that can support extended absences from work or family responsibilities is rare. Yet with a little planning, long periods of meditation can be incorporated into regular life. Physically, it might help you to work through aches and pains, ease tension and give you the energy to combat fatigue. Mentally, it can provide a way to escape from the maze of thoughts and find a deep sense of peace and clarity of mind. Extended meditation can enable you to become the calm observer of whatever you're thinking and feeling.

Arguably, these benefits grow exponentially depending on how long you can dedicate to the practice. But wellbeing and mindfulness instructor Hanna Milton stresses that regularity is more important than time. Brief but consistent will be far more effective than extended but sporadic practice.

Mindful pauses
To begin with, try to carve out short spells at least a few times a week when you can practise mindfulness, whether it's meditation, yoga or tai chi. If possible, build up to a daily routine, as this could help to sustain the benefits. The next is to extend the sessions. Hanna suggests gentle increments of maybe five minutes a week until you get to a length that feels right for you. 'This might change over time, or even from day-to-day,' she says. 'In my own practice, I have days where a shorter meditation is all I want and need.' Extended meditation is beneficial when it's a natural evolution of your practice and doesn't feel forced. The idea isn't that it becomes another chore to add to a to-do list. The time span should always be manageable. Hanna points out that 'if an hour-long session fills you with dread and you spend the whole time waiting for it to be over, you're not going to get a lot out of the practice'.

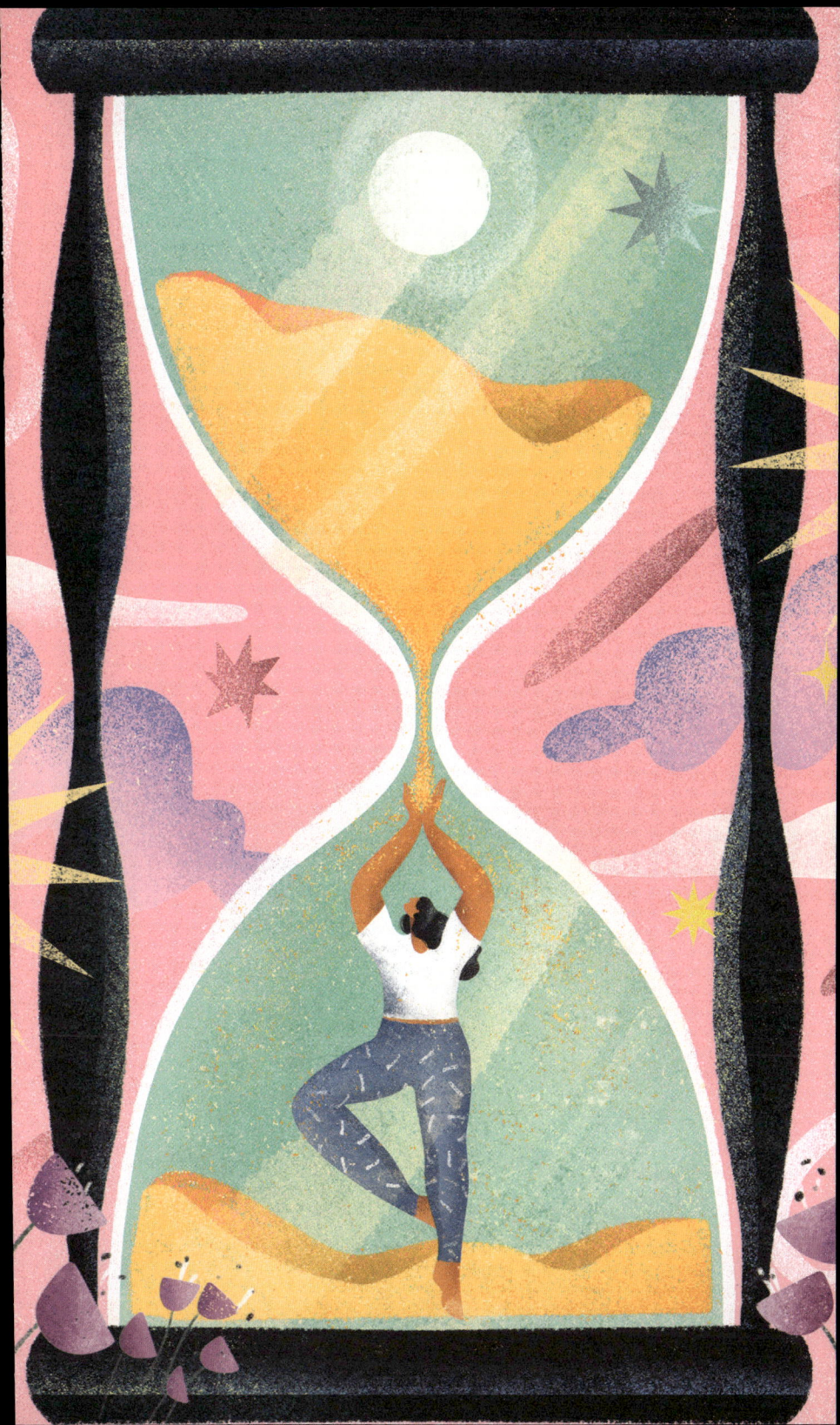

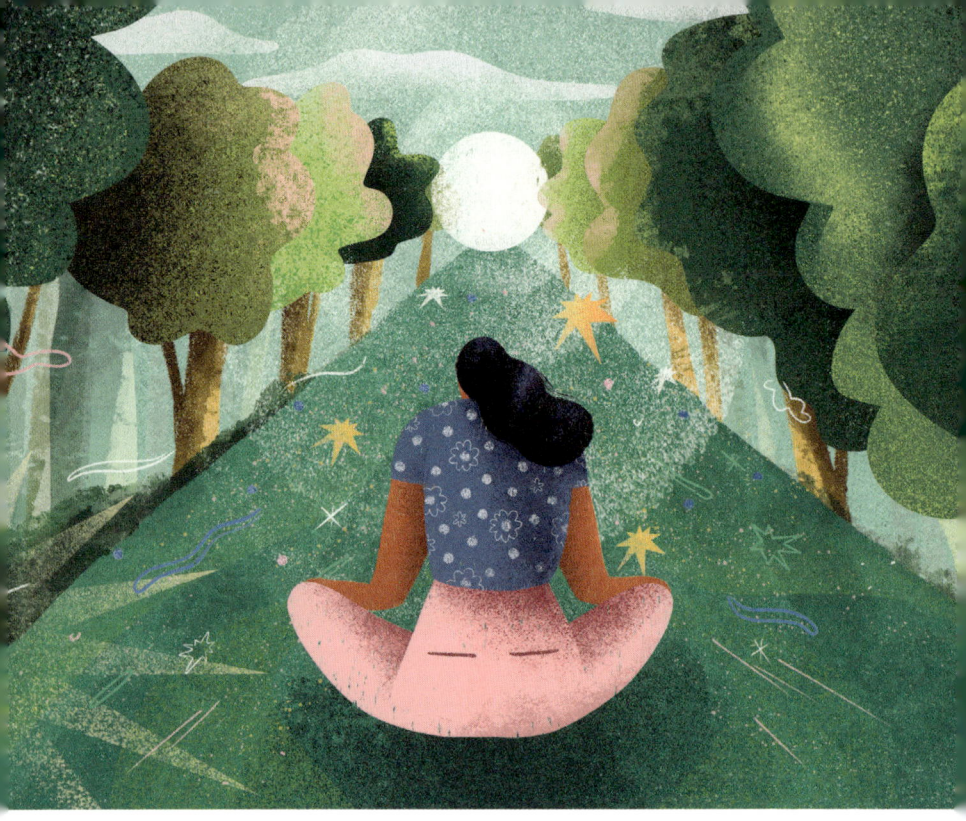

A fresh perspective

Buddhist tradition certainly indicates that it's important not to force yourself to meditate for longer periods or to get hung up on how much time you're setting aside for your practice. It is, after all, about being present in the moment, which is the opposite of what's referred to as striving – seeking a material or end goal. Starting a session with the thought you're not leaving the cushion for one hour might see you focusing determinedly on the clock until you've notched up your 60 minutes. This is likely to mean you become disconnected from the sensations in your body and less aware of your breathing. One way to counteract this is to notice any feelings of striving, let the thoughts drift by and then bring the focus back to the present.

The period of meditation is, of course, also dependent on how much time you have available. But if you find yourself thinking you just don't have a spare hour, you could try to look at it from another perspective. It might be, for example, that an extended session helps you to think more clearly and increases your productivity for the day, or you could even discover it means you need less rest. A 2010 study by the University of Kentucky, carried out in Delhi, India, looked at sleeping patterns of seven regular meditators, who practised for two or more hours daily, compared to 23 control participants. They discovered that, on average, the practitioners slept for 5.2 hours per night whereas their non-meditating counterparts needed 7.8 hours.

Unexpected challenges

Longer sessions can, however, pose challenges beyond time constraints. The process of going deeper into the mind can bring up strong feelings, both physical and mental. When considering the former, Hanna suggests asking yourself if you can feel relaxed about the discomfort: 'Listen to your body, if it doesn't feel right, don't do it,' she says. 'Move around and stretch between sessions, or try some yoga poses.' Sometimes being still and present with mild pain can help to release it, but there will be occasions when it's better to move around or end the meditation.

Psychologically, you might find strong emotions, including anger and sadness, swim up to the surface during stillness. This can be surprising when you've entered the practice hoping to find calm and to feel relaxed, but it's completely natural. The brain has myriad coping mechanisms for storing emotional traumas and sometimes the action of being present can unlock buried or repressed feelings that you might have been unconsciously avoiding, or that felt too painful to bear. Doing things that ground you in physical reality after a meditation session can help. Routine activities such as walking or housework can ease your transition back to your day. For some, crying or releasing these feelings might be as much a part of the healing process as sitting and noticing breaths.

Of course, long meditations won't be practical or work for everyone. That's totally fine and there's no need to worry. Instead, try harnessing your full attention and awareness to everyday activities, as well as pastimes. This will increase and lengthen the mindful moments in your day, almost an extended practice in itself. And ultimately the benefits of meditation are seen when they are interwoven into daily life. As Haikuin Ekaku, a Japanese Buddhist from the 17th century, said:

'While yet you live, practise meditation. Do not meditate only in a dark corner, but meditate always, standing, sitting, moving and resting. When your meditation continues throughout waking and sleeping, wherever you are is heaven itself.'

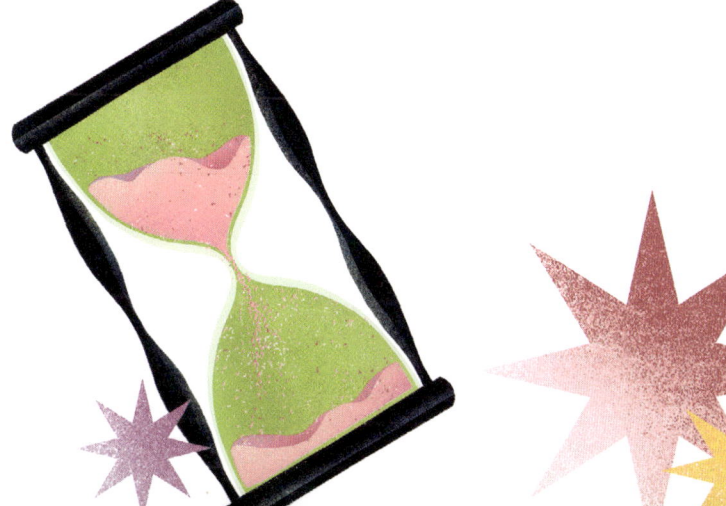

FIND YOUR BREATH

How to ease into your practice:

- Sit comfortably in a room or area where you won't be disturbed or distracted.

- Breathe naturally through the nose and bring conscious awareness to the breath, without trying to fix or change it. You might notice your breathing pattern naturally relaxing and deepening as the meditation continues, but don't try to force it.

- Notice the sensations that come with each inhalation and exhalation out of the nostrils.

- Continue to breathe through the nose. After each full in- and out-breath, count to 10. If you lose your place, return to one. This can also be reversed, so that the counting takes place before the start of each in-breath.

- If your mind wanders (it likely will do, many times), consciously try to stay present, notice your thoughts and return to your breath, then continue counting.

- When ready, come out of the meditation by slowly opening your eyes and being still for a moment. Gradually reacclimatise to your surroundings.

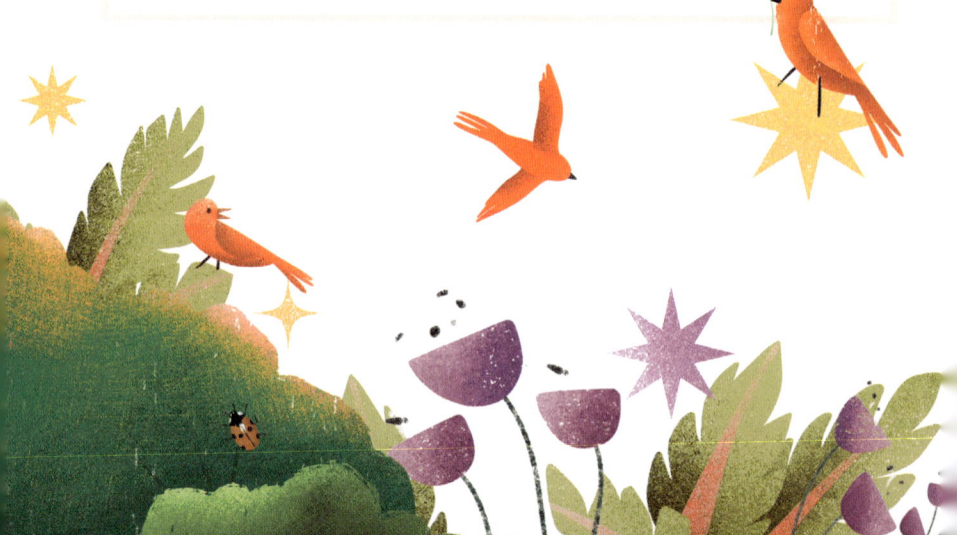

PUT EMOTIONS INTO WORDS

Professor of psychiatry at UCLA Dr Daniel J Siegel coined the phrase 'name it to tame it' to explain how articulating emotions can help people to cope with strong feelings. Journalling can be an effective way to explore thoughts that come to the fore during and after a practice. Use the space here to jot down anything that comes to mind.

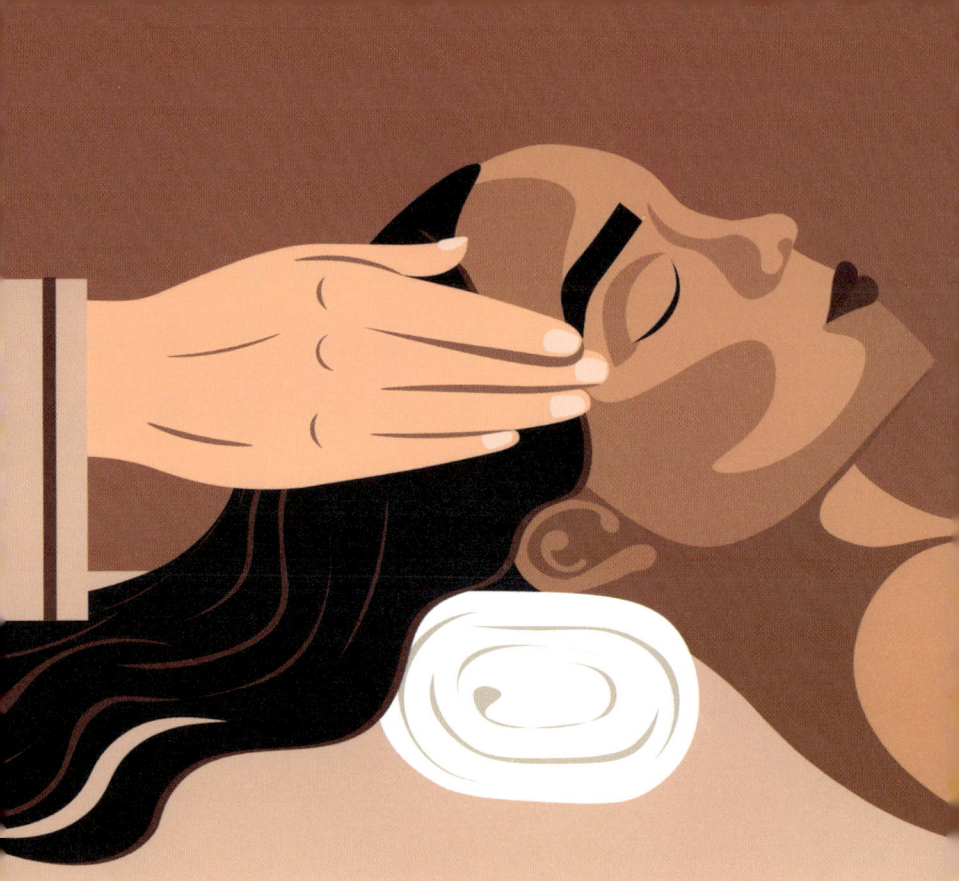

Ahead of the curve

Practised for thousands of years, Indian head massage promotes far more than just relaxation. Find out more about this ancient therapy and why it's head and shoulders above the rest

Though it may seem like a relatively recent concept in the west, head massage dates back more than 5,000 years to early Indian traditions. Ancient Ayurvedic texts say that, when used in conjunction with herbs, spices and aromatic oils, massage has an important medical function and cannot only 'strengthen muscles and firm skin', but also encourage the body's innate healing energy.

An integral aspect of Indian culture, massage is one of the first experiences a baby will have, as from birth to the age of three it's traditional for infants to be given a daily oil massage to 'keep them supple and in good health', while also encouraging bonding. This often continues throughout childhood.

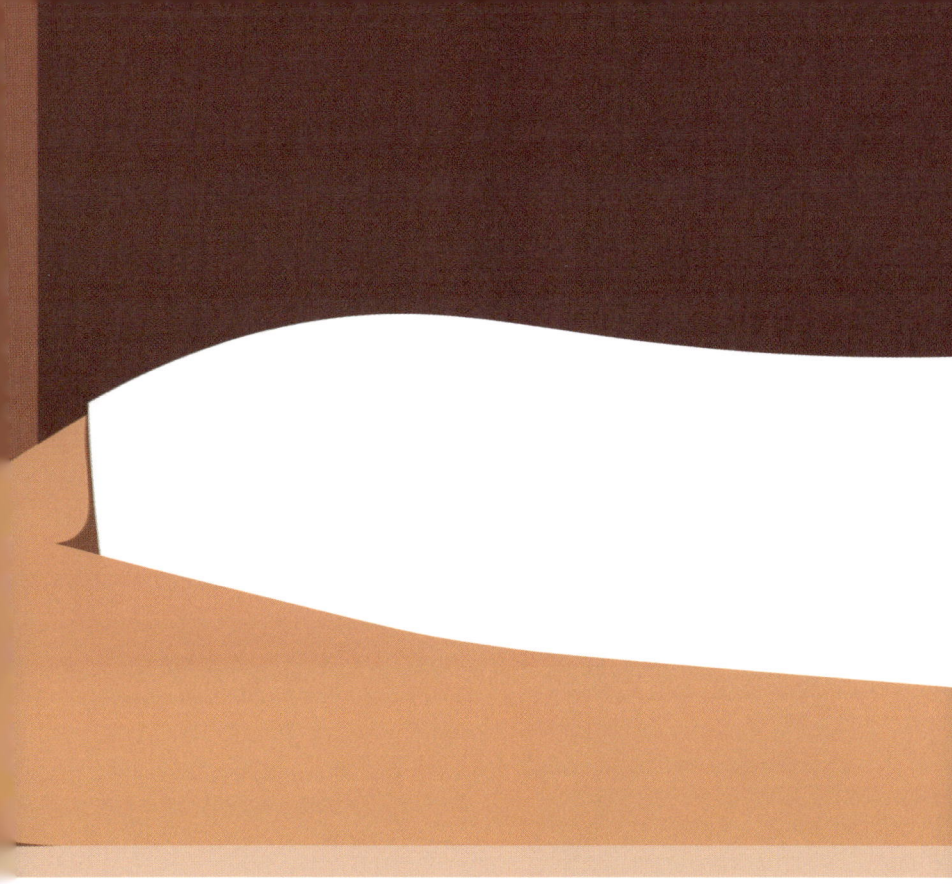

Deeper connection

For London-based counsellor Aisha Mirza, 30, Indian head massage has been a regular part of family life over the years, something shared between daughter, mother and grandmother. Aisha says: 'It's a really beautiful expression of care and love to give someone else, but also yourself.'

Aisha believes that massage isn't restricted to just giving to others and can be a way to get in touch with the self, too: 'Sometimes we can feel alienated from our bodies and unsure how to connect to it, but you know what feels good for yourself better than anyone else and [massage] is just a practice for working that out.' And you don't need to have special training: 'Massage is very intuitive, so checking in with yourself and experimenting can get you pretty far.'

This practice isn't confined to the family household. Traditionally, barbers would offer their customers an invigorating scalp massage – or champi – as part of a haircut. Champi is designed to stimulate and refresh the individual and it's from this Hindi word that 'shampoo' is derived. Indian women would share regular head massages with natural oils, such as coconut, almond, sesame and even henna, to strengthen and beautify their typically long hair.

New beginnings

When Narendra Mehta arrived in England in 1973 to train in massage and physiotherapy, he was shocked to discover that the head seemed to be neglected, even in a full body massage. Having been blind since the age of one, Mehta had a heightened sensitivity to touch and missed the therapeutic value of regular head massages. He returned to India in 1978 to research the ancient art, studying it wherever it was practised – in barber shops, on street corners and in family homes. Combining the barbers' champi, the women's soothing hair massages and his experience of heightened touch, Mehta came to two conclusions:

1. The therapy could benefit by extending to include the face, neck, upper arms and shoulder areas that hold a lot of stress and tension.
2. By introducing an Ayurvedic element into the massage to include work on the three highest chakras at the crown (top of head), brow (third eye) and throat (communication), the body's entire energy system could be rebalanced.

From this, he developed Indian head massage as we know it today – or Champissage, thought to be a portmanteau of champi and massage. After he exhibited this holistic practice in 1981 at Olympia, London, it exploded in popularity, spreading worldwide and even becoming a well-established form of complementary therapy among health practitioners.

A typical session

Myriad muscles support the head, neck and shoulders. Stress, anxiety and other factors such as tiredness and dehydration send these muscles into spasm, with tension keeping them tight and knotted. Indian head massage can alleviate these symptoms by releasing those tight muscles and aiding blood flow and oxygenating them, and can also help with fatigue, insomnia, headaches, migraine, sinusitis, joint mobility in the neck and shoulders, and circulation. It can be used to maintain wellbeing and to practise self-care, recharging physical and spiritual energy centres, or chakras, which are considered the focal point of prana – vital life force and energy.

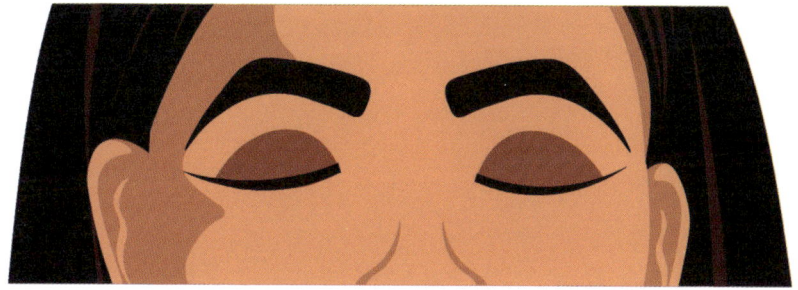

INDIAN HEAD SELF-MASSAGE ROUTINE

Whether you want to alleviate a headache, sleep better, stimulate hair growth or even just relax generally, here's Aisha's routine for massaging yourself:

You will need:
- Oil – use any whose scent you enjoy, such as coconut, almond, jasmine or even olive.
- A vest top/bare shoulders – optional, but it's nice to have skin-to-skin contact.

Things to remember:
- Experiment with different pressures and speed throughout to see what works for you. Do you want light, feathery touches or more firm movements?
- It's suggested to do each side separately, so your whole awareness is fixed on one point.
- Swap sides whenever you're ready to.
- For each side, either use the same hand or the opposite side's, whatever feels comfortable. If your arm gets tired, you can always support it with the other or rest your elbow on a surface.
- You can do any of the steps for however long you like, linger on one, omit another – it's all in your hands.

1. Start with a light meditation to get into the body. Close your eyes and bring awareness to your surroundings, your senses and your breath. Take a minute to send some gratitude to your lungs and your body.

2. Take three deep breaths, in from the nose and out through the mouth. Try to extend the duration of each breath. Do a whole body scan, imagining a laser of awareness going from your toes to your head. Keep your awareness on the head, relaxing your jaw and your face and allowing everything to be heavy.

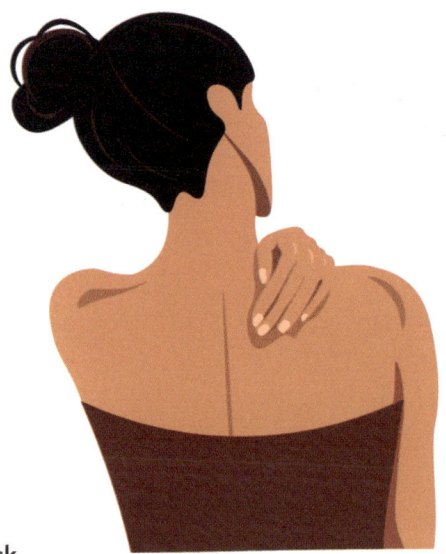

Shoulder/back

3. Rub some oil between the hands and start rubbing your shoulders, using one hand at a time on the opposite side.

4. With two or three fingers, go from the top of your spine upwards and at some point you'll feel a little ridge at the bottom of your skull. This is the occipital bone, Aisha says: 'It's a nice place to get accustomed to finding on yourself and others as it can work as an anchor when you're doing this kind of work. If you don't know where to start, try from here – it's important as it holds the head up.'

5. From one side, at the occipital bone, move the fingers in a circular motion towards the heart. Move the fingers to about halfway down the neck. Then go from the occipital bone in the same way, this time to the bottom of the neck, top of the shoulder blade.

6. To work the trapezius, follow the same line, this time with a dragging motion with four fingers, going from the occipital, down the back of the neck, across the top of the shoulder blade, ending with a little flick to 'flick out the tension'. Then reaching as far back on your shoulder blades as is comfortable, drag your fingers forward, flicking the tension off in front of you this time.

7. 'Pluck' each side of the shoulder muscle, grabbing it upwards with your whole hand and then letting go in a short, sharp pincer-like movement.

8. Bring the hands down the side of the face, extremely slowly and lightly, just barely brushing the skin. Bring them down to the bottom of the neck then place them on your chest.

Scalp

9. Rub some more oil into the hands and then into the hair, as liberally as you like, working it into the scalp. After the massage is over, ideally leave this oil overnight in the hair to soak in and really nourish it.

10. Curl your hand into a loose, soft C-shape and place on the temple. Move it in a circular motion, paying particular attention to how you respond to it. Move your C-shaped hand in the same motion to the occipital, then slowly across the back of the head, towards the hairline.

11. Repeat this pathway with circular motions but with a claw-shaped hand instead. If you're pregnant or have epilepsy, be aware this can be quite stimulating.

12. Give your whole scalp a rub, you can use the palm of your hands to do this if it feels good. Remember to keep breathing and relax your jaw.

13. Using the pincer motion from Step 7, pluck the head with both hands.

14. Move around the head using a 'raindrop' motion with the fingers (again, this is quite stimulating).

15. With a loose, soft chopping motion, start 'hacking' across the scalp.

16. If you have long enough hair, scoop it all up, above the crown chakra at the top of the head, holding it with one hand above the other. Breathing in, pull the hair upwards, and when breathing out, let go.

17. Repeat Step 8.

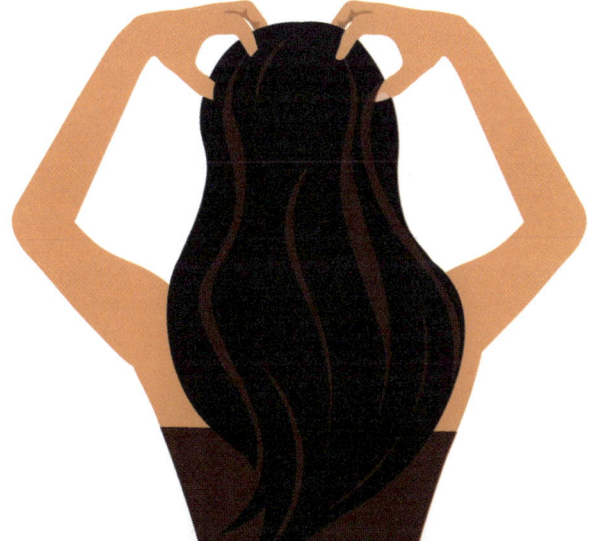

Face

18. Feel free to wash your hands at this point, you can use a different oil or a moisturiser for the face if you wish. With two hands, starting from the third eye, move up to the hairline and across to the temple with two/three fingers in little circular movements.

19. With a dragging motion, go from your third eye, across the brow bone, to the temple. Then, from the temple, move across the cheekbone towards the nose with the little circular motions.

20. When you reach the nose, place two fingers on each side of the nostrils, and drag the fingers slowly and deliberately under the cheekbones. This will help with any sinus issues.

21. This will bring you to the top of the jaw, which holds a lot of tension. Use the circular motions to work the jaw, to the chin, under the lip. Then when you're ready, massage the ears and their backs with the circular motions, ending with a pull on each lobe.

22. Repeat Step 8, then take three deep breaths as at the start, breathing out all the tension.

23. Make sure to drink water after your massage.

To learn more about Indian head massage, find a practitioner or training course, visit champissageinternational.com.

Indian head massage is not suitable for everyone. If you have epilepsy, neurological conditions such as MS, any form of arthritis affecting the neck, shoulders and upper arms, conditions such as osteoporosis, cancer, diabetes, aneurosa, high or low blood pressure or may be pregnant, it is essential to seek medical advice beforehand.

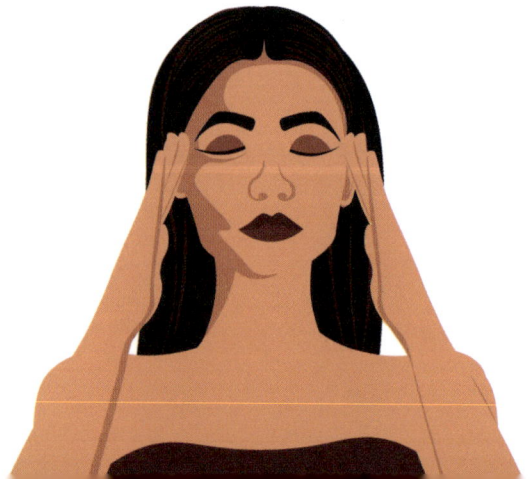

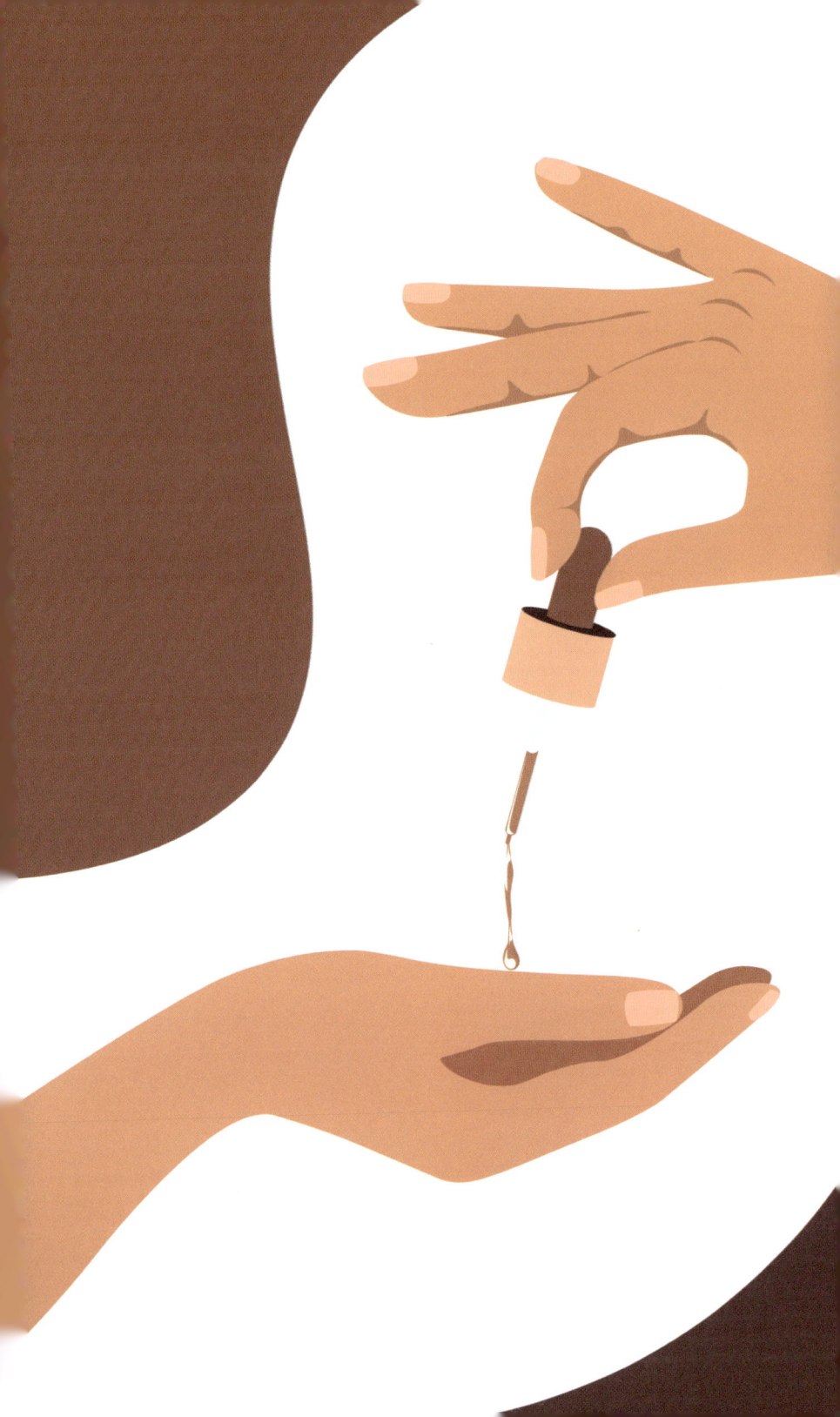

Discomfort zone

During meditation, it's possible to focus your attention and escape the jumbled thoughts that may be causing you stress. But what if, far from being bad for you, a modicum of stress can help you feel good, achieve goals and grow as a person?

Stress – there's plenty of information out there on the negative effects that too much tension can have on your body and mind. But what if an entirely stress-free existence turned out to be far from ideal? In fact, what if it wasn't desirable at all? Clinical psychologist Lisa Damour is well aware of the harm that stress can cause when it's chronic or traumatic. Lisa, who has a practice in Ohio, US, defines chronic stress as 'stressful events that persist without a break', while trauma is 'an overwhelming, harrowing event'. But outside those responses, she believes that stress is a 'growth-giving part of life'.

Embracing the uncomfortable
Psychotherapist Amy Morin agrees: 'Sometimes, people want to eliminate all stress from their lives, but some stress is good for us.'

For one thing, small amounts of the stuff can create a powerful resilience by building a person's ability to tolerate discomfort. This is important, says Lisa, because being 100 per cent happy and calm all the time is an impossible standard to meet. 'It's problematic to suggest that [good] mental health should be defined as feeling calm and relaxed all of the time. That is not possible, necessary or even healthy,' she says. 'Instead, we should define mental health as having the right feeling at the right time and being able to manage it effectively.'

Even a traditionally happy event, like getting married or bringing home a new baby, can present stressful moments. However, embracing a small amount of discomfort can help people prepare for whatever the future holds. And trying things that are slightly stressful can ultimately help a person achieve their personal and professional goals.

'Doing uncomfortable things can help us sharpen our abilities – such as our emotion regulation skills,' says Amy. 'For example, when you're in an uncomfortable situation, your brain might tell you to quit or you might think the anxiety you're experiencing is a sign you can't succeed.

'But when you keep working towards your goal, despite those feelings, you build mental strength. You prove to yourself you're stronger than you think and you'll develop confidence that you can handle bigger challenges in future.'

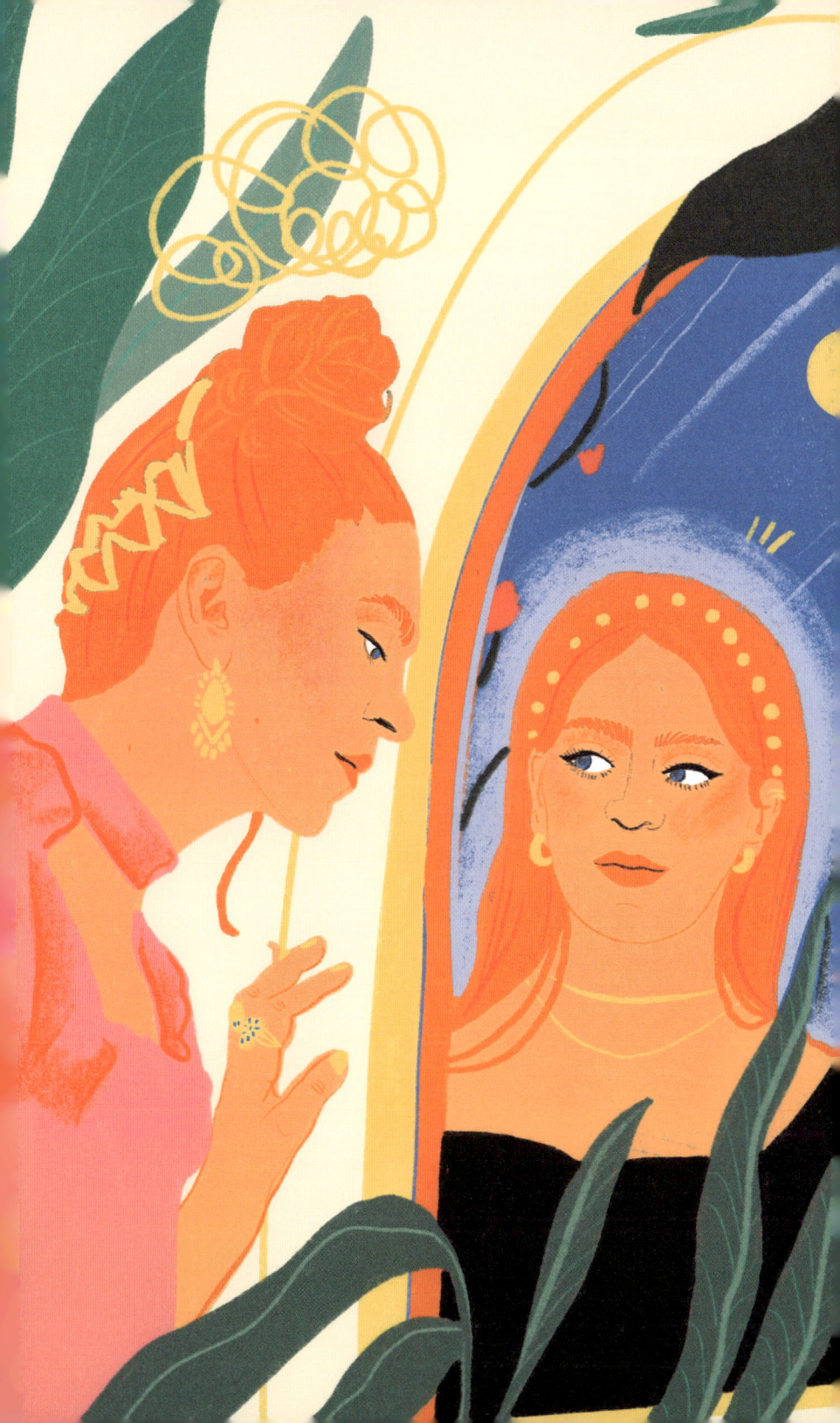

Building mental strength

Caleigh Breen, 30, a hairstylist in Calgary, Canada, learned this first-hand when she opened her own salon. As a self-confessed introvert with mild social anxiety, she found the self-promotion that was necessary for her business to thrive quite stressful. 'It goes against some of my core instincts, which are to stay in the background and not have any of the attention on me,' she says. 'But when you run your own business you have to force yourself to be comfortable being out there, especially nowadays when social media is such a core part of marketing.' Facing her fears made Caleigh realise that she was her own worst critic. 'Every time I've been nervous to put myself out there, I've just decided to do it and see what happens. Each time I did, I've been met with overwhelming support.'

She says being bold and not letting social anxiety call the shots has built her mental strength and resilience. This and other stressors that come with being a small-business owner have taught her that 'every time I come up against a hurdle and solve it, the less likely I am to run away from it'. Caleigh has also learned that she performs 'a lot better' under pressure. 'With a small amount of stress, I suppose I'm thinking more consciously about my clients, making them feel comfortable and listening to their needs. Maybe it's because I'm trying to create a calm atmosphere to lower my own stress.'

A little of what you don't fancy...

This tallies with a psychological principle called the Yerkes-Dodson law, which states that stress can improve performance, up to a point. 'We actually perform a bit better when we're in a heightened state of arousal – at least to an extent,' Amy says. 'A little anxiety will get your heart pumping and make you more alert so you might do better than if you had no stress at all.' She warns, however, that there's a tipping point: 'Experiencing too much anxiety can put you in such a heightened state of alert that you can have trouble thinking and difficulty responding in a helpful manner.'

Reframing the way you think about stress has been shown to intensify its positive effect on performance. Harvard researchers put 50 study subjects in a situation designed to get their hearts racing and palms sweating. It involved being evaluated on their public-speaking skills, followed by a tricky test. Ahead of their speech, some of the participants were told to ignore the stress they felt. Others were given no instructions and played video games while they waited. The remaining participants were told about the positive impacts of stress and how physical responses like a pounding heart had evolved to help boost how humans function in difficult times. Compared to the other subjects, the speeches from this last group were rated as better and they appeared more confident – they even smiled more.

Little by little

Exposing yourself to healthy stress doesn't mean diving headfirst into pressurised situations or biting off more than you can chew. It's important these challenges lie just outside your comfort zone, and it's crucial to take existing commitments into account – so it probably wouldn't be wise for someone already working 60-hour weeks to take on another big volunteer project. The best way to add healthy stress to your life is to do something that makes you feel 'some mild discomfort', says Amy. This will vary from person to person. Some might baulk at the idea of meeting new people while others might be anxious when faced with a workout routine. She says: 'When you discover something that you avoid doing because it's uncomfortable, that's what you want to tackle.'

A 2013 study in the journal *Psychological Science* found that trying things that challenge you can be good for your brain. The researchers found that older people who learned new skills, like quilting or photography, experienced a bigger mental boost than those who did stimulating but familiar tasks, such as listening to classical music or solving word puzzles. They concluded that the enhancement zone, where peak learning happens, lies just beyond the comfort zone. Lisa agrees that it's helpful to push past what feels comfortable. 'People experience stress any time they're working at the edge of their current capacity – also a time when we tend to expand that capacity,' she says. 'When an individual can weather the stressful event, they come away from it more capable and resilient.'

Stretch for the positive

According to Amy, new challenges help people to learn about themselves, others and the world, and can help challenge self-limiting beliefs. 'You might consider yourself to be unintelligent, clumsy or socially awkward, for example, but challenging yourself to do new things can help you see those labels aren't true.' She says the best source of healthy stress, whether social, emotional, physical or financial, is doing something that stretches you in positive ways. 'Creating new challenges for yourself could help you build the mental strength you need to reach your greatest potential.'

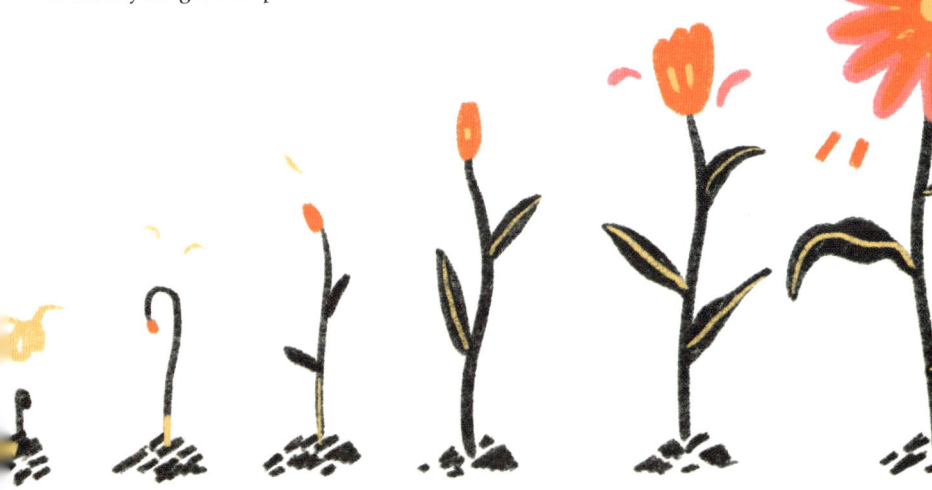

POSITIVE STRESS CHALLENGES

It'll be different for everyone, but the right challenge will feel a little difficult. Here are a few suggestions:

- Shake up your morning routine. Wake up a little earlier than usual and make your bed right away.

- Stretch yourself socially. Reach out to five people a week to say hello.

- Flex your finances. Try cutting out online shopping for one month, and see how much you can save.

- Set a fitness goal. Train for a 5k run or an obstacle race. Or buy a pedometer and set a target of walking 10,000 steps every day for a month.

- Fight public-speaking fears. Offer to lead a meeting or give a presentation to a small group at work or socially. Or give a short toast at a family event or a friend's birthday dinner.

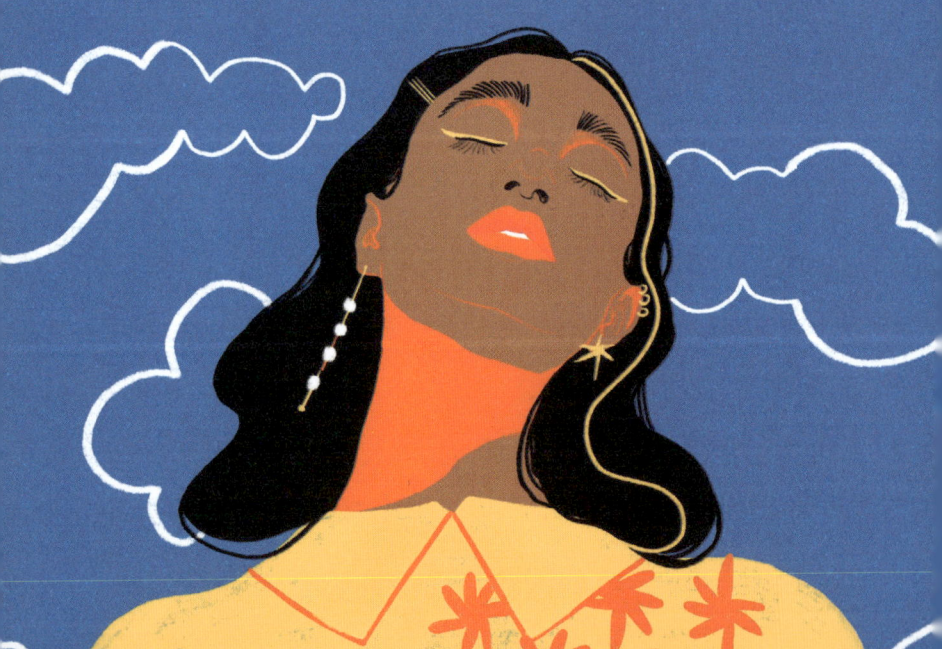

HARNESS THE POWER OF HEALTHY STRESS

If you're struggling to decide what might work for you, or you'd prefer to design your own healthy stress challenge, ask yourself these questions:

Which situations make me uncomfortable?

....

....

....

....

....

....

....

....

What have I been avoiding that could add value to my life?

....

....

....

....

....

....

....

....

What self-limiting beliefs do I hold? How could I challenge them?

....
....
....
....
....
....
....
....
....

In which areas do I need to build mental strength?

....
....
....
....
....
....
....
....

Have there been challenging situations in my past that led to growth? How were they helpful?

> 'Take rest; a field that has rested gives a bountiful crop'
> Ovid

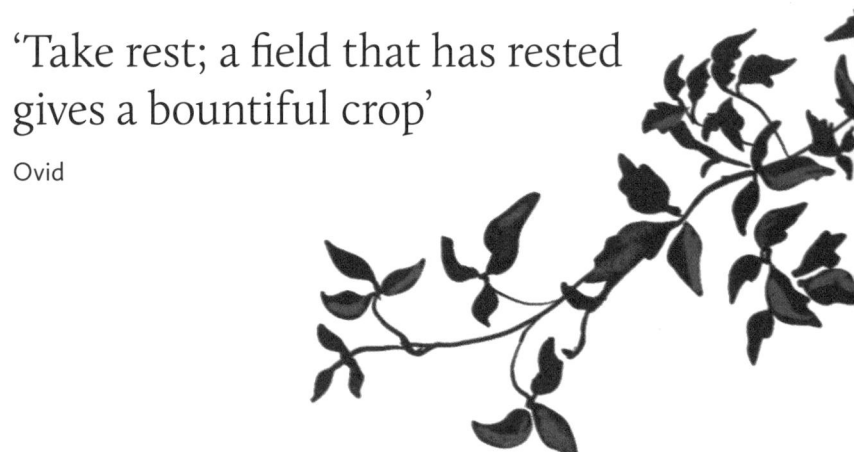

DIY wellness weekend

A wellbeing sabbatical needn't break the bank or involve a year away from home. Here's how to make three days really work for you and reap the benefits for months to come

Evidence suggests that people who take extended time off tend to live longer and are happier, in both their personal and work lives. But taking weeks, months or even a year out on a costly programme of treatments and downtime is rarely practical (or affordable). A more manageable way to re-evaluate your lifestyle might be to incorporate a three-day, home-based wellness sabbatical once every three months, or even annually, allowing you to stop, take check and focus on your needs.

Bhavya Arora, transformational life and career coach, explains: 'Escaping a busy life to spend three days to focus on growth and empowerment is all it takes to reboot. It's enough time to leave everything behind. Me-time is not a myth, it's real. So, drop any guilt… only you can make it happen. Set an intention of how you would like to feel at the end of your break and what you would like to achieve mentally, emotionally and physically. You'll be surprised at what you can achieve in this time.'

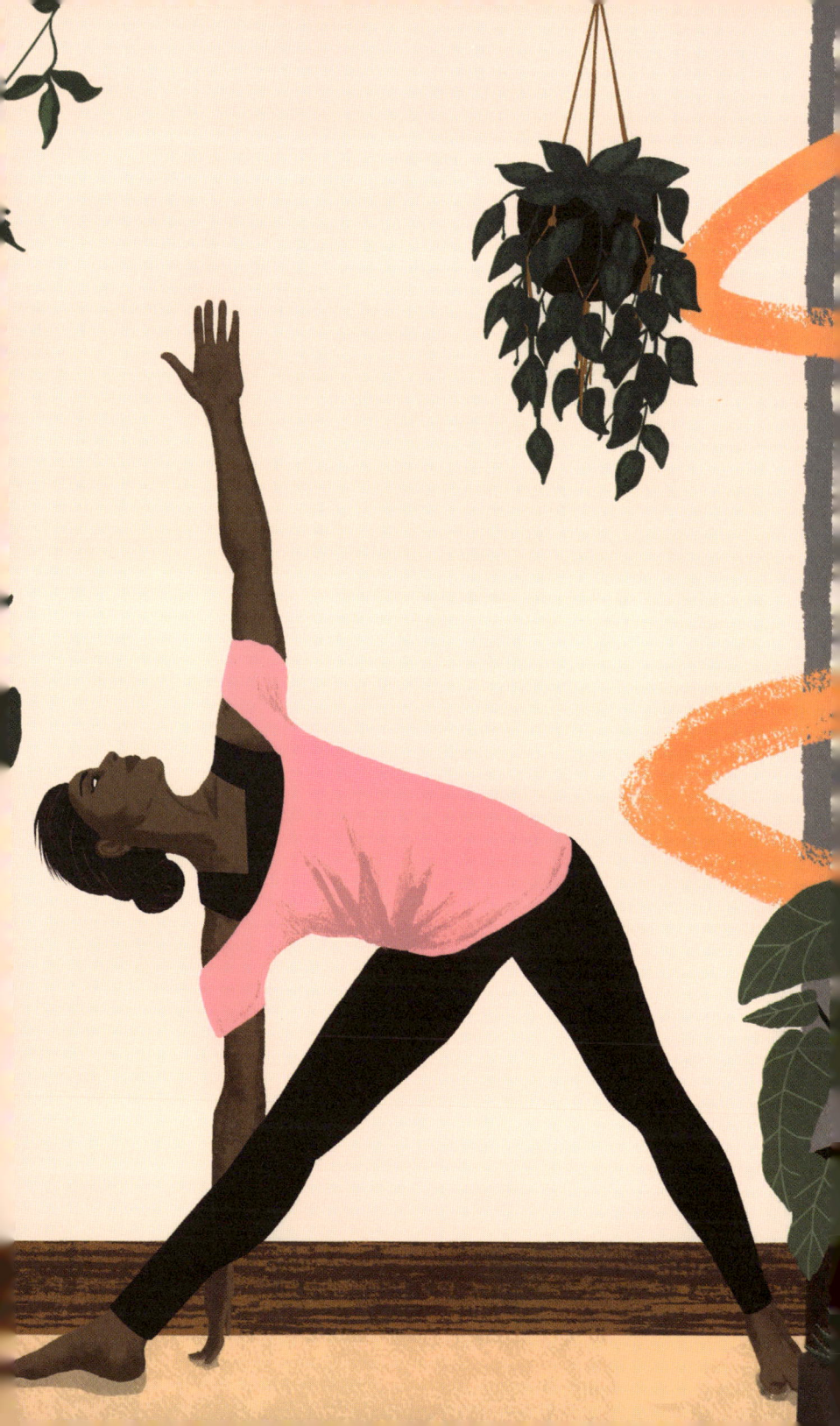

Reasons to retreat

How do you know when you need to take a sharp exit from the daily grind? There are several signs, but common ones include:

- You just need a break.
- Life feels like hard work.
- You feel confused about your direction.
- You're feeling overwhelmed by your to-do list.
- You're feeling worried or uncertain about the future.
- Life doesn't feel fulfilling, as though something is missing.

If this sounds like you, begin with some research about how you will spend your three days. You don't have to take them next week or next month. You might choose to wait six or eight months. But it's important to use your time wisely, so you can make the best choices for yourself and determine exactly what you'll benefit from the most. Start by making a list of as many healing and wellness experiences you'd like to try or ones that have previously worked for you.

These can include in-class or online kundalini yoga, dancing, Zen meditation, time in nature, a different sleep routine or simply human connection. You might also consider stress-reducing treatments that are new to you, perhaps shiatsu massage, reiki or acupuncture. Think of areas that might open up new doors of possibility.

Relax and reboot

When it comes to your three days, you might choose to place yourself in a beautiful, natural setting. Depending on the time of year (and size of your garden), you could set up a cosy tent and kit it out with some of your favourite things. Alternatively, create a special environment indoors, perhaps a room just for you.

What's important is to be able to experience and internalise how it feels to find a level of clear thinking and creativity that's present in a relaxed state, something that's hard to tap into when life's busy or stressful. The aim is for this to inspire and sustain you long after the sabbatical.

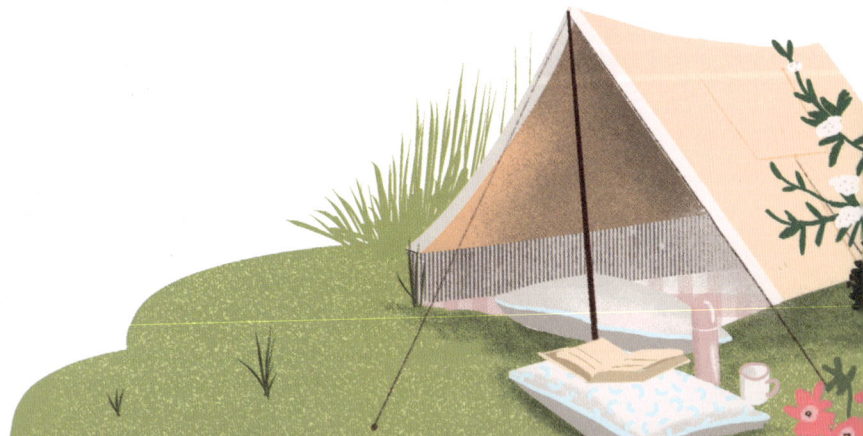

JOURNALLING TIPS

Ahead of the sabbatical, it can be useful to engage in writing exercises that enable you to reflect on and explore thoughts, and define your needs. Here's two you might try:

1. Make a list of your fears, beliefs, dreams, hopes, goals and things you'd like to do before you reach your next birthday.

2. Spend six minutes writing a letter to the 'You' of the future – maybe in one or five years' time – telling yourself what brings you joy, who's in your life now and how it's different to yours in the future.

BEFORE YOU BEGIN

1. Set boundaries
Sort out any chores and routines beforehand. If possible, try to be home alone. See if a partner, family members or flatmates could spend the time at a friend or relative's house. If this isn't practical, establish boundaries and set a clear rule – do not disturb me.

2. Make your environment Zen
Candles, aromatherapy, relaxing music, herbal tea, whatever they are, stock up on and arrange your favourite things. Wherever possible, have nutritious pre-made meals to hand and don't forget any essential movie-night accompaniments.

3. Choose your stationery
Find a notebook or journal to jot down your thoughts and reflections as they come to you.

4. Plan any classes or get-togethers
If permitted, book a massage, try a reflexology session, attend a yoga class, go to the gym or meet up with a friend.

5. Limit screen time
Other than an online yoga, fitness or meditation session, allow a maximum of 30 minutes a day for gadgets and only use it to check for essential messages. It's not for work or general social-media scrolling. Let friends know what you're doing and silence any notifications that might prove distracting.

6. Explore different options
You could rewrite your version of success and then use it to reconnect with your purpose and values in life, deciding what truly matters to you and if you want or need to have a healthier lifestyle, physically, emotionally or psychologically. If so, how might you achieve this?

TODAY'S THE DAY

Everyone will have their own idea about their optimal environment and schedule for their sabbatical. The following is a possible timetable – tailor it to suit your personal needs

7.45am A cup of tea in one hand and a book in the other, followed by a short run, walk, cycle or even an online fitness session.

9am Breakfast of fresh fruits, oats and maybe eggs at home, or nip out to a café and watch the world pass by while you eat.

10am Window shopping, browsing, study of local architecture or maybe a mindful walk.

11am A relaxing bath followed by journalling and reflection about feelings, emotions, likes, dislikes, wants and goals. Nutritious lunch to follow.

1.30pm Post-lunch nap, meditation or body-scan exercise (visit breathemagazine.com/body-scan).

2.30pm Post-nap gratitude exercise – three things to feel grateful for in life.

3pm Massage or treatment, either at home or somewhere local. If this isn't practical, you could try an Indian head massage (*see page 16*).

6pm Pump up the music, get cooking or head out for a meal.

9.30pm A moment of reflection, looking at new insights, observations, hopes, needs, dreams and things that could be done differently.

10pm Create affirmations based on the desires and hopes identified while journalling. Recite them before going to bed at a reasonable hour.

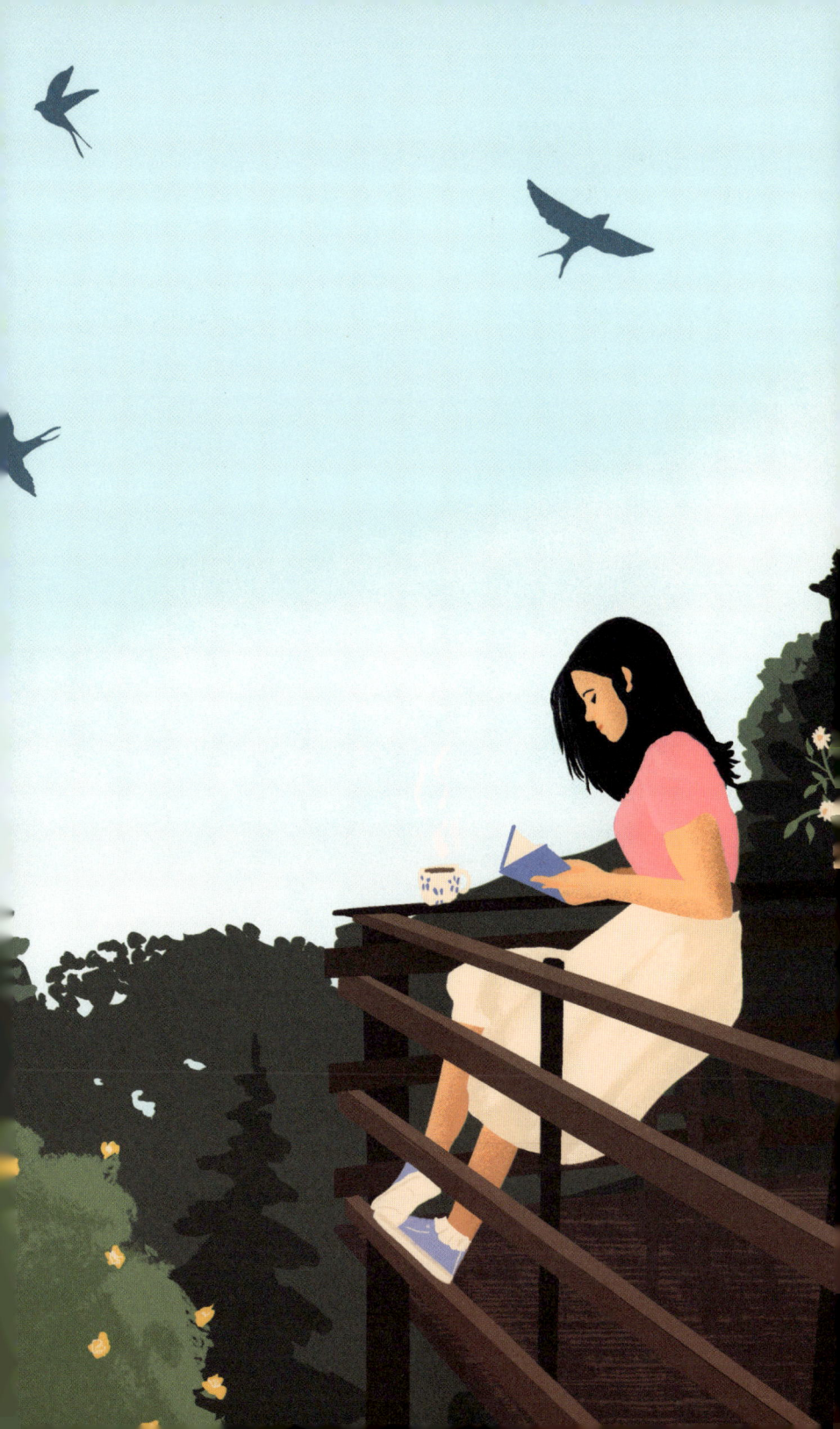

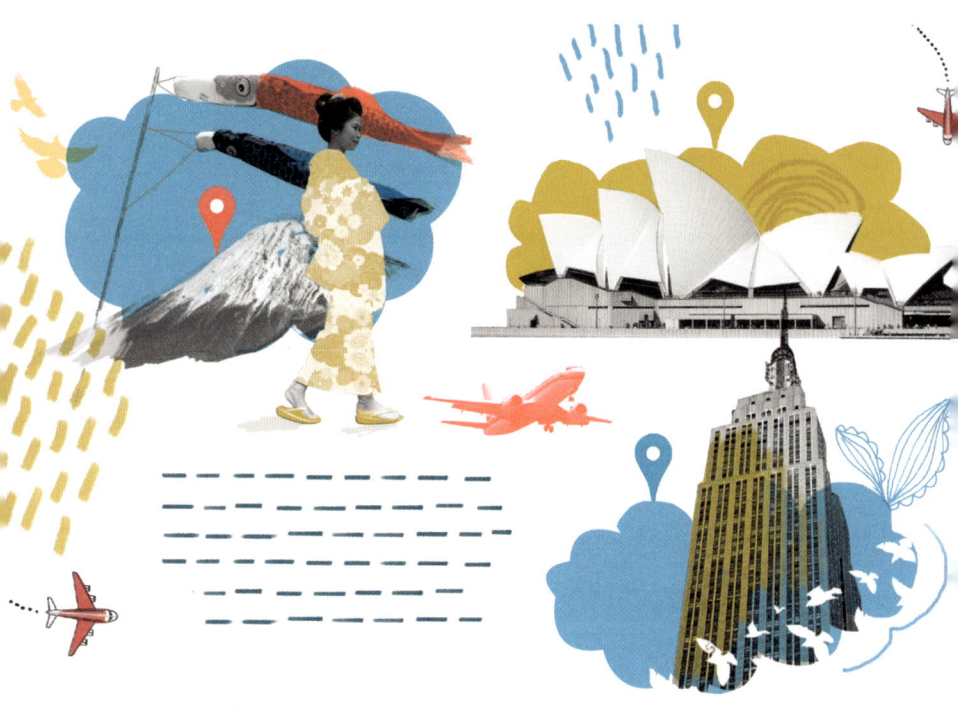

Manifestly for you

Can committing to good deeds as part of creative visualisation help to make your dreams a reality?

Have you ever made a vision board? Sometimes known as dream boards, they're a relatively common concept, involving creating a visual representation of goals, inspirations and dreams that can be pinned somewhere within easy eyesight as a constant reminder of your intentions. Some people like to design a vision board on a computer or via a site like Pinterest, while others love to get creative with art supplies and pictures clipped from magazines. The end result tends to be a colourful board that can be hung somewhere to inspire you daily.

What if you took the project even further – pledging good deeds and charitable actions, investing positive energy as you work towards your dreams? That's where a manifestation board comes in. Manifestation boards are similar to vision boards, but in addition to your dreams and aspirations you include pledges of altruistic actions you're going to take. It shifts the focus to giving as well as receiving, sending positivity out into the world as well as calling it back to yourself. You could think of it as generating good karma or maybe even a reminder of 'the bigger picture'.

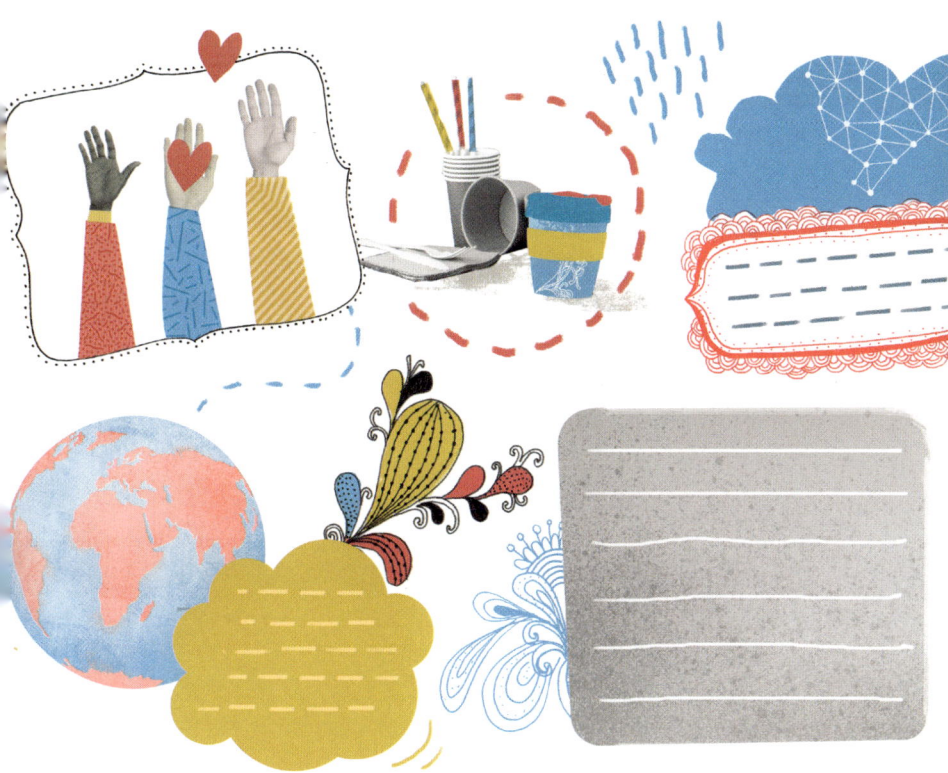

Drilling down

The simplest way to create a manifestation board is to divide your pinboard or document into two pieces. The first half can be treated as a traditional vision board, where you visualise your goals and dreams. They might include relationship, friendship or financial goals, career or business ambitions, family hopes or health and wellness aims. The key is to be really specific and give yourself a vivid image to focus on. For example, if one of your dreams is to travel, it's more useful to include photos of the actual destinations, buildings or cities you'd most like to visit rather than generic beach or mountain shots.

The second half of your board is where you commit energy to manifesting your dreams by pledging good deeds or actions. Again it's helpful to be specific, so rather than deciding you want to save the oceans it might be better to make a pledge to start buying shampoo bars or stop using plastic cutlery. You can include anything you like here – and remember to use your unique skills.

So if you're good with kids, you could decide to volunteer with a scout troop. If your career involves finance, you could offer to do the books for a local charity or community group. Alternatively, you might decide to do one daily random act of kindness. The idea is that your manifestation board is equally weighted, so for every dream or ambition there's an altruistic counter pledge.

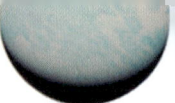

Leading your subconscious

Manifestation, vision and dream boards all work by tapping into the power of visualisation, a technique used by psychologists, life coaches, athletes and business people. Seeing is believing and visualisation is a form of mental rehearsal. Olympic athletes have been using it for decades to improve performance. If you hang your board somewhere where you'll see it often, such as above your desk or kitchen counter, then you're effectively creating a mini-visualisation exercise every time you look at it. When you ask yourself who you want to be, or what kind of a day you want to have, you have a visual answer to hand.

There's a famous saying: 'If you can dream it, then you can do it.' According to a research paper on visualisation published by the International Coach Academy, it works by imprinting your goals and dreams onto your subconscious mind, which operates using pictures and visuals, and runs 90 per cent of your life. Visualisation and exercises like vision boards help programme your brain to work towards achieving your goals.

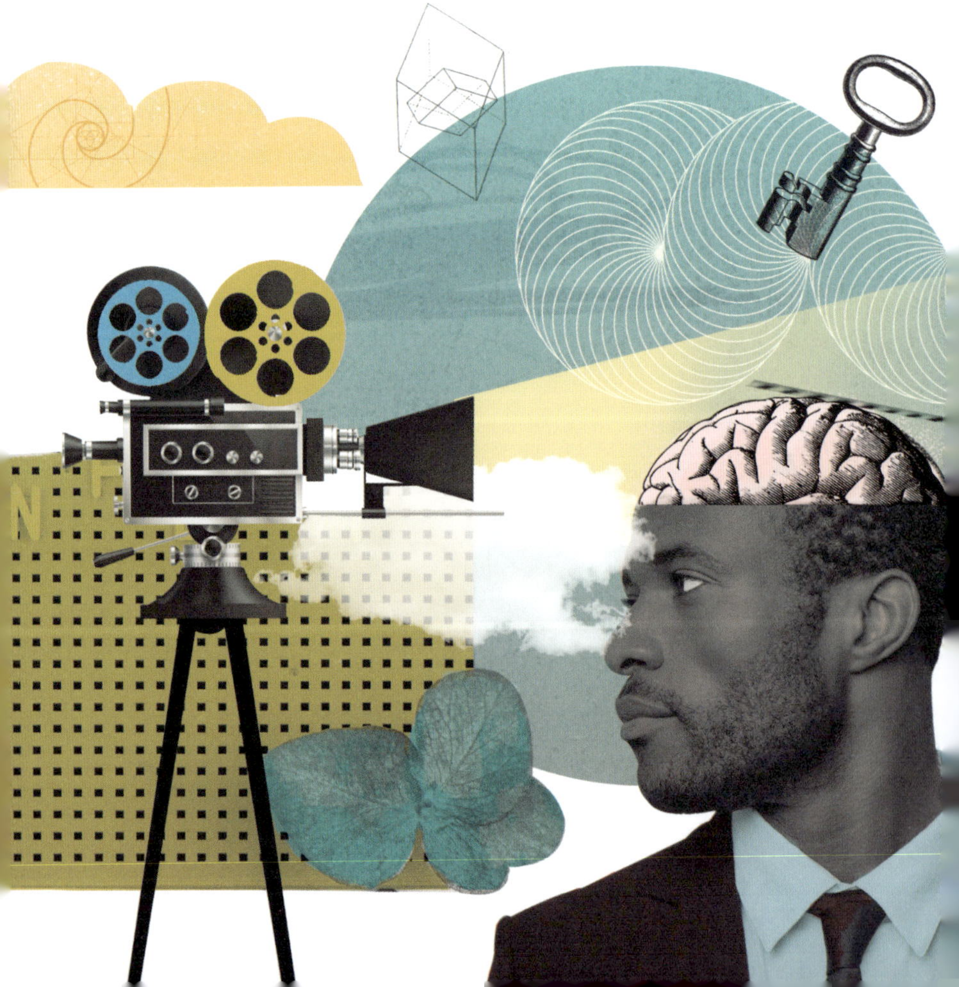

Tapping into altruism

Creating positive energy by pledging good deeds on a manifestation board makes the exercise even more powerful, according to Scottish psychic medium Carol McGee. She's used manifestation boards to build a successful business and financial security… and even claims to have manifested movie star Brad Pitt in her village of Erskine. Carol's first manifestation board, created back in 2011, featured her dream car, a white Audi TT, financial stability and a villa in Cyprus. In return she pledged to raise funds for a local charity, Golden Friendships Clydebank, and offer free healing sessions and readings to nearby churches and community organisations.

Almost a decade later Carol owns her white Audi TT, has built a successful mediumship business and spends part of every year working in Cyprus. She's also raised thousands of pounds for charity. But perhaps her most surprising success involved Hollywood royalty. She explains: 'I wanted to put a wildcard on my board so I printed a photo of Brad Pitt and said I wanted him to come to Erskine. It's a tiny village on the outskirts of Glasgow… hardly an A-list hangout, so I thought it'd never happen. But just a few months later an item on the local news stopped me in my tracks. Brad Pitt was filming a movie called *World War Z* in Glasgow and he was staying with Angelina Jolie and the kids in a 5-star hotel, a couple of hundred yards from my home. What are the chances of that?'

Carol says manifestation boards appealed to her because of the feeling of 'giving back'. She adds: 'Traditional vision boards struck me as being a bit too self-centred. By pledging the charity work and fundraising I felt I was creating good karma and positive energy, and focusing on the world outside myself too. Giving and helping people are such powerful things.

'My only regret is that I wasn't more specific about that Brad Pitt visit. I should have visualised him popping round for a cup of tea!'

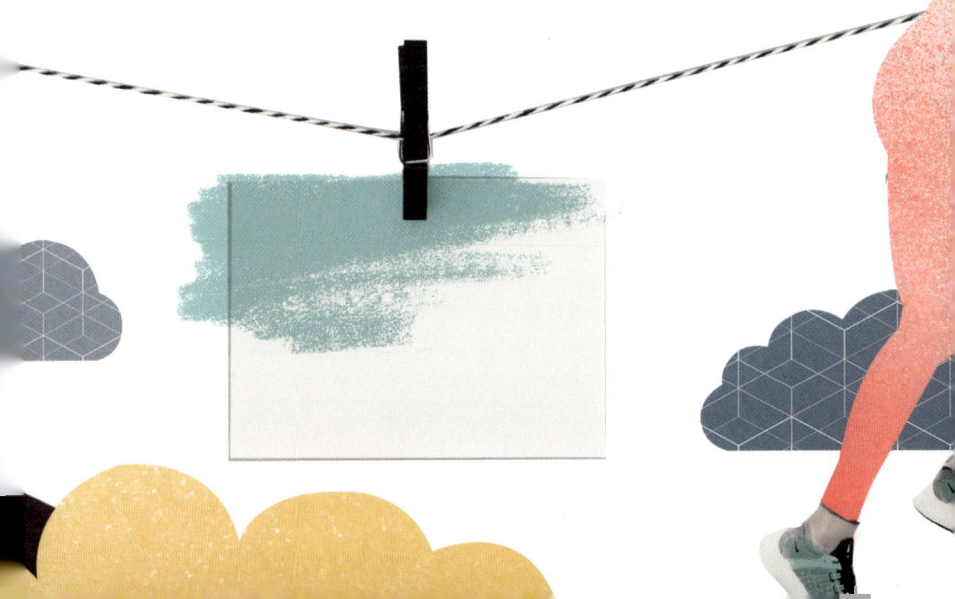

HOW TO CREATE A MANIFESTATION BOARD

1. Make it a positive experience
The idea is that it's inspiring and fun, so try to find a time to do it when you won't be rushed or disturbed and can give it your full attention. You might like to light candles or play your favourite music. Dream big and get your creative juices flowing.

2. Gather your materials
If you're making it by hand, you'll need a pin- or corkboard, colourful pens and a stack of old magazines to cut photos from – or pictures printed from the internet. If you're doing it on a computer, you'll need access to images or a tool like Pinterest, plus a printer to run off the finished product and frame to display it.

3. Think about what appeals to you visually
Are you inspired by photographs or illustrations, words and quotes, or would you like to include pictures of people you admire? Do you prefer a computerised or homemade look? Be as creative as you can – you could even add certificates, postcards or ticket stubs.

4. Be specific
Visualisation works best when it's detailed. If you want more money, create an image of what your ideal bank balance would look like, or pension fund, or a monthly total. If you want to run faster, pin a hoped-for personal best time to the board, if you want to run further, set a distance. Meaningful personal images work best.

5. Make sure your pledges are achievable
Again it pays to be specific and think about what you can realistically commit your time and resources to. For example, instead of deciding you want to volunteer with children, pledge to give one evening a fortnight to coaching a kids' football team. If you want to freshen up mealtimes, you could start to observe meat-free Mondays. Do you have an older neighbour whose dog needs walking or a colleague who'd benefit from some mentorship? And how can you represent your pledges visually on your board to inspire you?

'Do not dwell in the past, do not dream of the future, concentrate the mind on the present moment'

Buddha

Open invitation

Why exploring honestly and fully your thoughts about mindfulness and meditation can help to establish and tailor a sustainable practice that meets your needs

Why do some people find mindfulness easier than others? Have you tried it, but felt it just didn't click with you? Did you feel resistance to the idea, or was it something else? You might have sat down eagerly on a meditation cushion, only to face the first of many distractions – outside noise or inside chatter. Maybe you felt unclear about why you were doing it or whether you were doing it right. The act of sitting still and observing your breath can feel alien at first, and a wave of fear, calm or irritation might follow. These are all perfectly human responses to noticing and being with your thoughts.

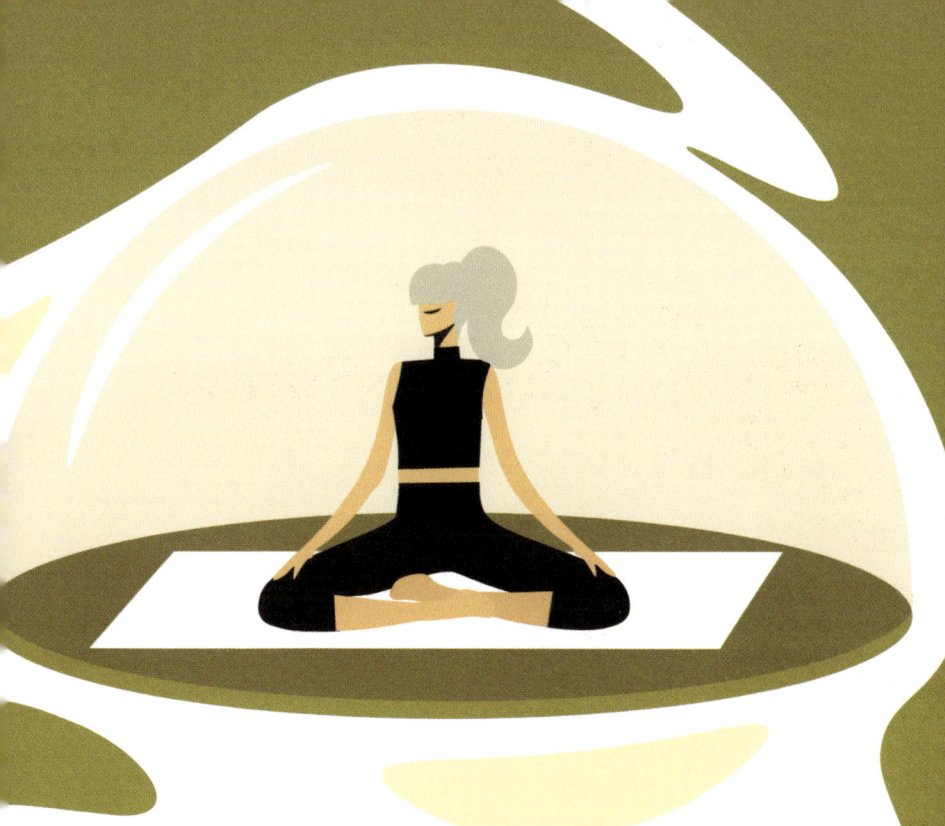

Learning to listen

Bringing awareness to and observing what is going on for you amid the noise, as well as beneath it, can be deep work. However, according to a 2010 study, if you can stick with it, mindfulness continues to be a compelling approach for reducing stress, anxiety, anger, chronic pain disorders, substance abuse, memory loss and trauma. The same research also shows that meditation can result in physical and mental health benefits after as little as eight weeks of daily practice.

Yet many continue to find the area challenging. One common idea is that distractions will disturb your practice, but let's face it, how many people live in a noise-free environment? Most mindfulness training explains how to work with sounds and unwanted or difficult feelings as a way to be mindful. Another misconception is that you have to clear your mind of thoughts to practise mindfulness, but this isn't the case. Mindfulness and meditation aren't about stopping all thoughts and entering a void of nothingness. They're about noticing thoughts as they arise. That doesn't mean you allow a train of thought to become a full narrative on what you need to do today. Rather, it's that the noticing might allow you to let it go before it gets a grip on you. Of course, the same thought, or a slightly different one, might pop up again in a few seconds, and that's okay – again, just notice it and let it go. At times, this helps the thoughts to pass, on other occasions, it might not. All this means is that during your mindfulness session a lot of thoughts came up, which is fine.

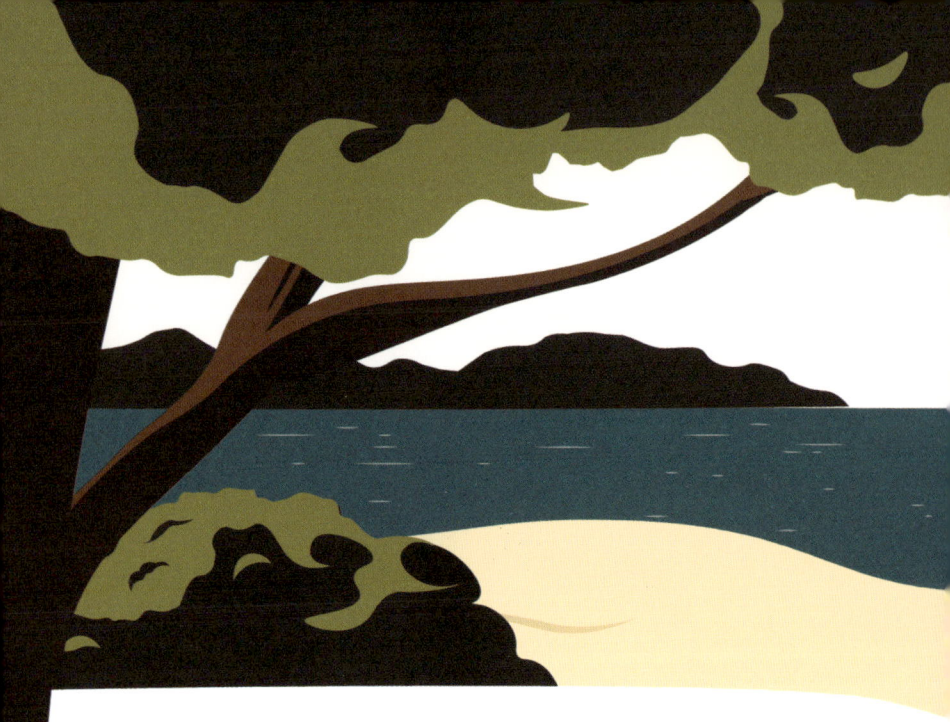

Be in the moment

To be fair, it does take practice and some days might feel easier than others. However, regardless of this, it's important not to judge the success of your practice. Part of mindfulness is just witnessing and accepting your experience for what it is, whether it feels like an easy or challenging practice on that day.

If you've revisited mindfulness several times and still find it difficult, you're not alone. Some people have found various techniques, such as app-based guided sessions, to be helpful. Kim Palmer, the founder of the Clementine hypnotherapy app, admits mindfulness was making her feel more anxious rather than less. She turned to hypnotherapy, which proved beneficial, and went on to create a hypnosis-led app of visualisation sessions that aim to relax, change patterns and support feelings of anxiety or stress. 'The concept of mindfulness felt completely unachievable to me,' she says, 'it was too much for my busy brain to comprehend and too big a hurdle. I tried it a few times, failed, and then the mental barrier went up, which made me feel like a failure. Then I tried hypnotherapy which was a total game changer.

'During my first session I was able to relax completely. I felt at ease and could surrender my mind to do whatever it wanted to do. Because I was able to let go and not feel any pressure to stop my mind wandering, I could tune into the powerful words and it felt amazing.' Kim now feels able to be more mindful in her daily life. 'I think [this is] because I've focused on finding moments in my day where I know I can experience a bit of joy. As an example, I'm even mindful when I go to the bathroom. I find I'm not rushing it, and I can even dream a bit while I'm in there. The same feelings can be applied when I'm cooking.'

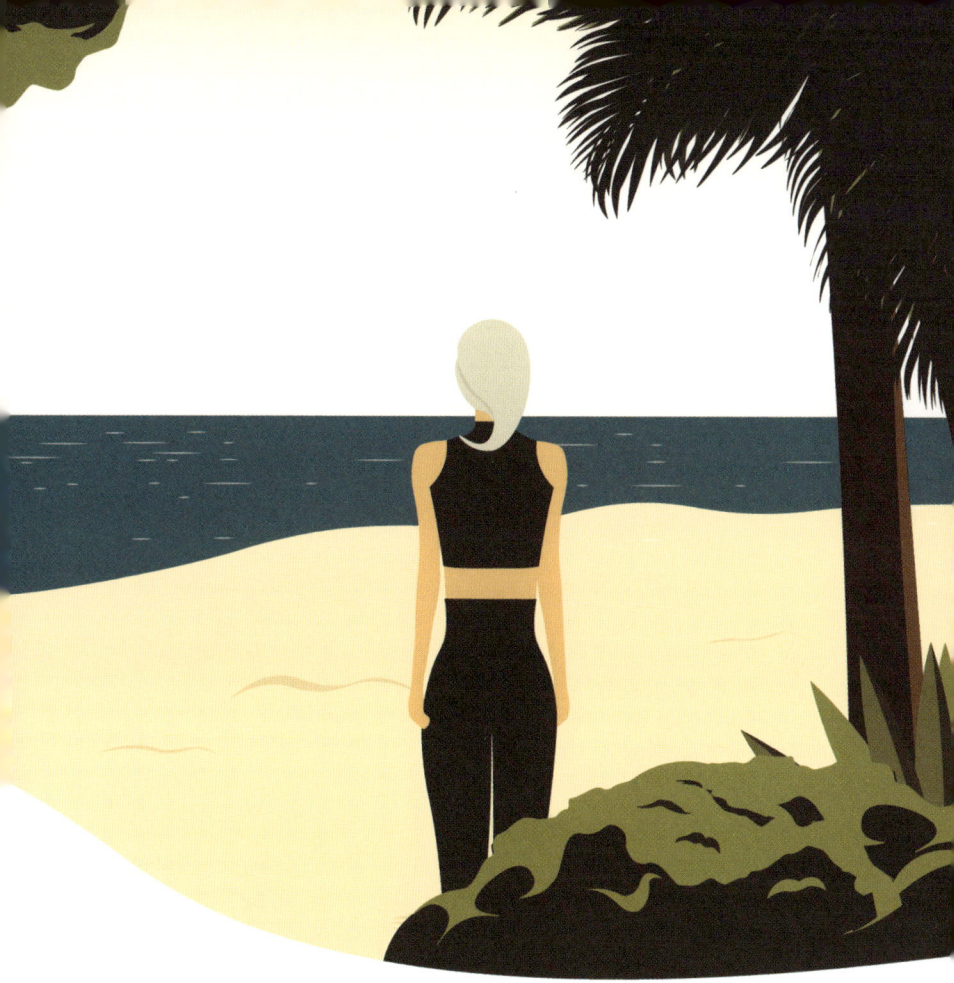

Recognise the positives
That's the beauty of mindfulness, it isn't just about sitting crossed-legged on a cushion for 20 minutes twice a day. It's important to integrate mindful moments into your day, and follow what resonates with you, which in itself is being mindful of how you feel and what you need at that moment in time.

If you've struggled with mindfulness or would like to rekindle a regular practice, you could approach it as you might physical exercise. If you think about it, jogging around your neighbourhood or lifting weights in your bedroom every day might not seem thrilling. Yet knowing you're doing it for a healthier and stronger body can help ease you through the arduous training. Similarly, if you learn to enjoy the process of mindfulness, and spend time developing your practice in the knowledge your mental health is becoming stronger as a result, you're more likely to stick to it longer term and be able to reap the optimum results.

MAKE IT PERSONAL

Tips for establishing a regular meditation practice and incorporating mindfulness into everyday life:

- Tune into why you want to practise mindfulness. Remind yourself of your motivation each time you feel yourself wandering away from it – and if you do, above all, be kind to yourself. You could begin with just 10 minutes a day and see how it goes from there. It might also help to dedicate a regular time each day to a session and put it in your diary as an appointment with yourself.

- Aim to become more aware of how you feel as you go about everyday tasks. This could include washing up, eating, walking, driving or taking a shower. In the process, you might find you become more mindful of sensations in the body, feelings and emotions present at the time, and thoughts and distractions. If you get lost in the distraction, there's nothing wrong with it, just notice the experience and come back to being fully present with what you were doing.

- You might have triggers to stop and notice where your mind is and come back to the present moment, knowing your body is in this present moment, not the past or future. These triggers could be turning on a light, going through a doorway, putting the kettle on, waking up in the morning or the time before you sleep at night.

- It's like turning up and being fully present in every moment of your waking life, whatever's happening – after all, the definition of mindfulness is knowing what's happening, while it is happening, whatever it is.

- For ongoing help, join a local mindfulness class with a teacher who resonates with you, and is registered with the British Association of Mindfulness-Based Approaches.

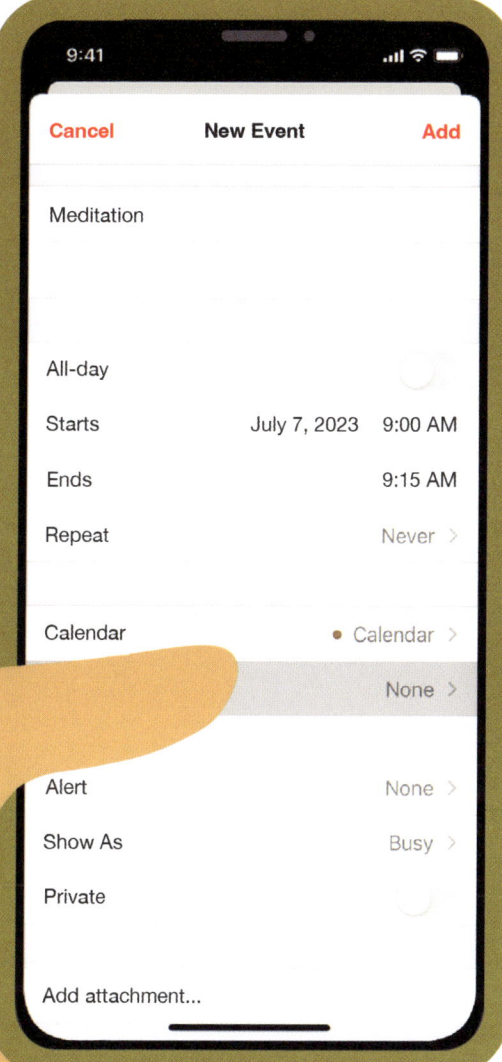

MIND MAP OF MEDITATIONS

There are many different forms of meditation, including Buddhist, guided and mantra, as well as non-secular mindfulness. Here are a few notes to help you choose which might be most effective for you

1. Mindful walking – for active and kinaesthetic learners
This is one way to incorporate a more active form of mindfulness into your daily life. It involves being consciously aware while you take walks around your environment.

2. Visualisation meditation – for creatives
This is a broad definition of a meditation or mindfulness session that involves an element of guided visualisation, usually narrated by an instructor.

3. Mindfulness meditation – an all-rounder
With its roots in Buddhism, this option has various forms, one of the main ones being mindfulness of breathing. It helps you to use your breath to anchor you in the moment.

4. Loving kindness meditation or skilful compassion visualisation – for cultivating compassion
Also with origins in Buddhism and other spiritual practices, these meditations involve sending love to yourself, to others and to all living beings.

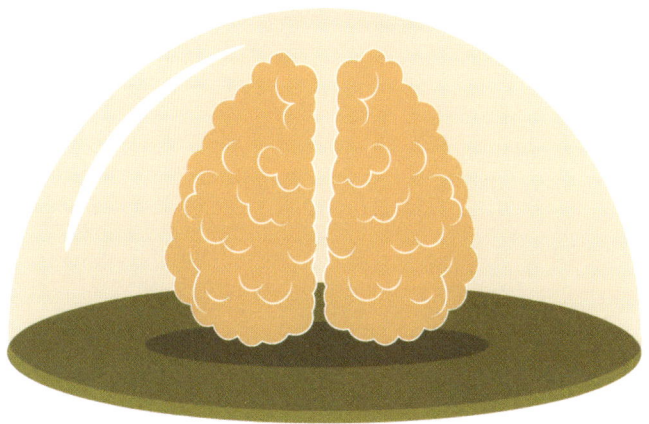

5. Zen meditation – for practitioners looking for something new
Stemming from Japanese Buddhism, the goal here is to regulate attention. It's sometimes known as a practice that involves 'thinking about not thinking'.

6. Transcendental meditation – for those who want to use powerful mantras
Adapted from the Vedic meditation tradition of India, and developed by Indian spiritual figure Maharishi Mahesh Yogi, this involves the use of a personal mantra, and is practised for 20 minutes twice a day with the eyes closed.

7. Vipassanā – for seasoned practitioners looking to go deeper
This focuses on a type of mindfulness of breathing technique combined with the contemplation of impermanence (that is, all things are impermanent), as a way to gain insight into the true nature of this reality.

8. The body scan – aids sleep
Also known as progressive muscle relaxation, this is usually done lying on your back as you slowly relax each body part, moving gradually from your head to your toes. See breathemagazine.com/body-scan for an example.

WALK THIS WAY

Tempted to try conscious movement? Find time today to take a 20-minute stroll and follow this simple exercise:

Walking is one of the nation's most popular exercises, according to Sport England. But rather than allowing your mind to wander and start to think about what you'll watch on TV tonight, use this mindful exercise to get the most from your walk instead.

- Walk at a natural pace, breathing fully and deeply, and pay attention to every step you take. Place your hands wherever it's most comfortable – by your sides, on your belly, behind your back. Try not to let them swing, or they may become a distraction.

- Notice the subtle movement in your legs and be aware of how your feet touch the ground and keep you upright. Feel how each foot swings ahead in turn and how the heel hits the ground – then the ball, then the toes.

- Notice the rest of your body. Does it shift from side to side? Feel the bend in your knees as you walk. Become aware of the muscles in your calves.

- After a short while, shift your awareness to the sights and sounds around you. Engage your senses and take a deep breath in through your nose. What can you smell? What can you see? What is moving? Is there a breeze? With each thought, simply acknowledge it, and then let it go.

- Return to the physical sensation of striding ahead and note how you're feeling mentally and physically in the present moment. Has your breathing changed while you've been making these observations?

Practise this purposeful movement often, alongside other conscious exercises, and you'll be left feeling strong, empowered and invigorated.

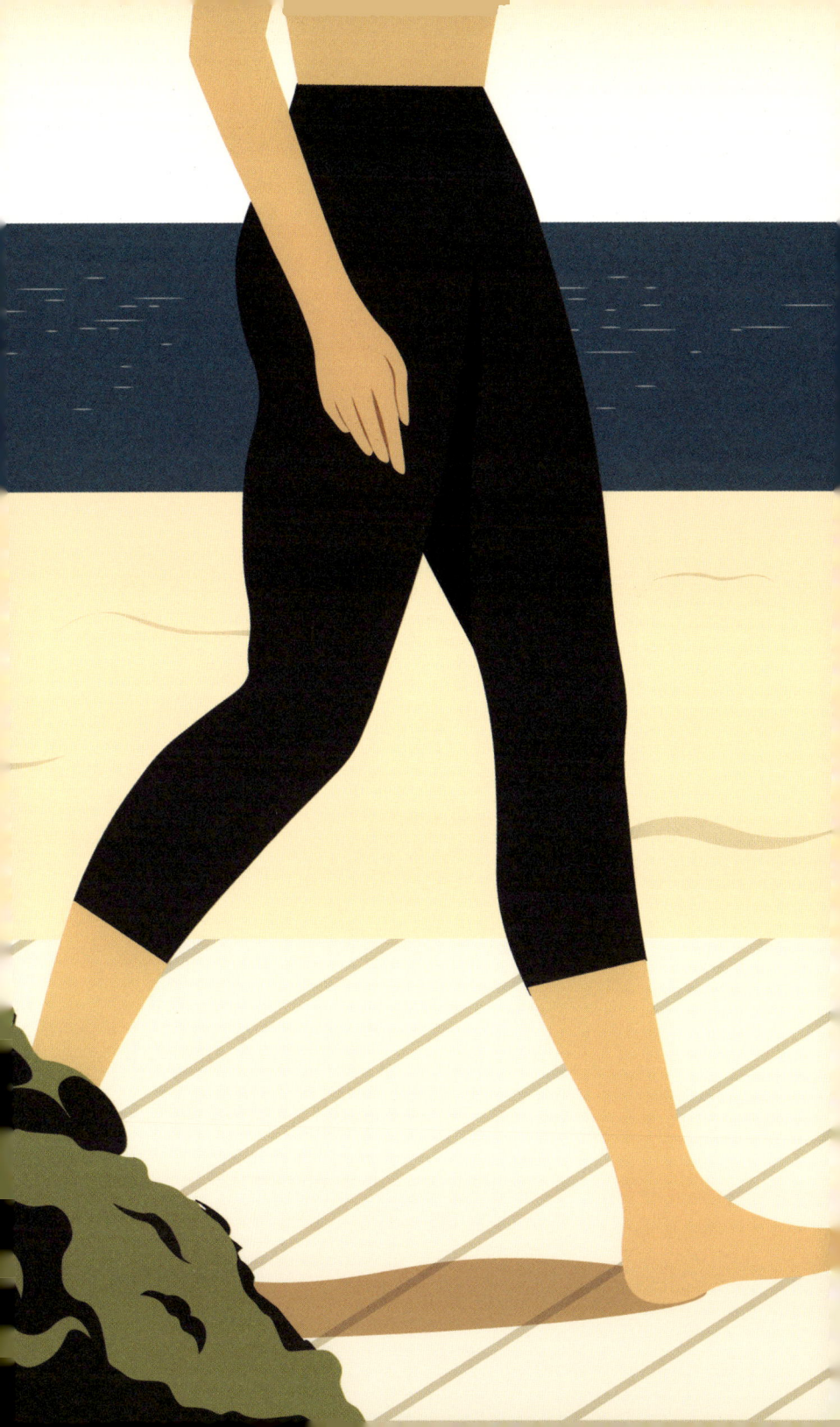

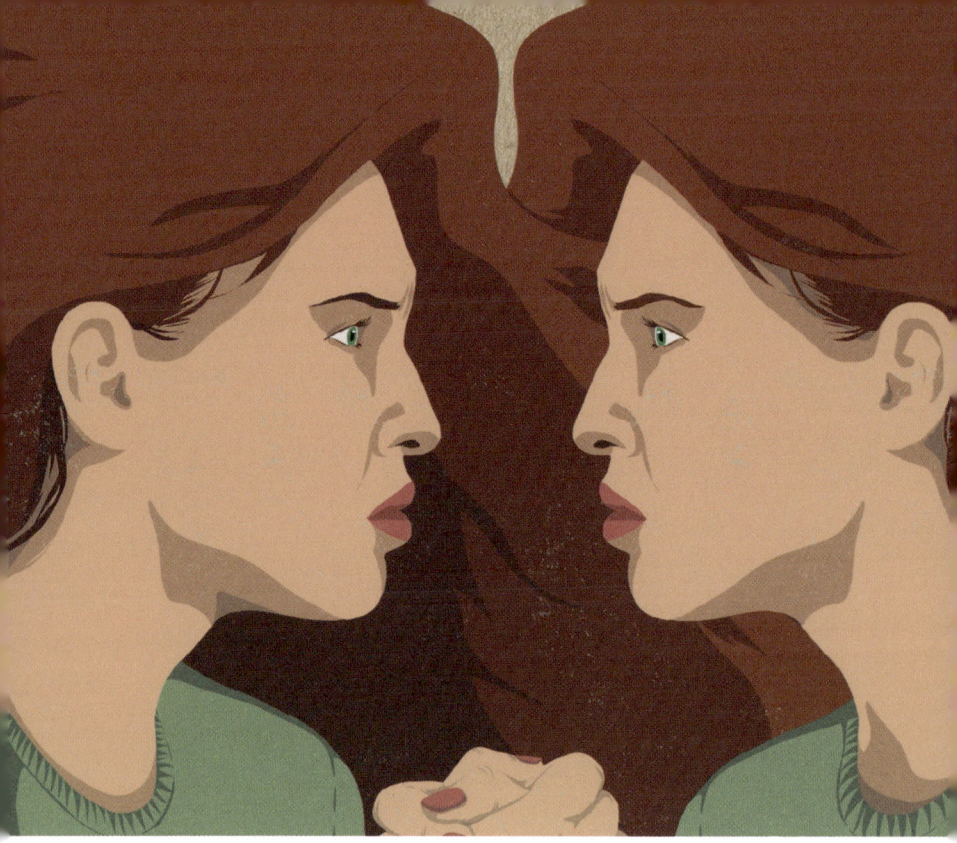

Parts of the story

Meditation can be a useful tool for keeping the ego in check, but whether it's fear and confidence or doubt and belief, there are times when our different states collide. Understanding why this happens can lead the way to resolution

People comprise different parts. These include roles such as friend, parent, gardener, runner and colleague. They also entail varied characteristics, including a desire to learn new things, to relax, to be level-headed or be a little wild.

Parts are sometimes referred to as ego states. This concept, which stemmed from the work of neurologist Sigmund Freud and was taken up by other pioneers in the field, has been developed by professor Gordon Emmerson, founding director at Resource Therapy International in Melbourne, Australia. He explains how individuals are 'made up of an ego family of states. You are… a number of different states; each has its own feeling of power, weakness, emotion, logic or other personal traits'.

Conflicting views

Ego states, which are a normal function of the psyche, are usually created in response to a new experience, frustration or trauma. 'Most start in childhood,' says Gordon, 'and as the repertoire of states increases, fewer are formed in adolescence, and fewer still in adulthood.' These states or parts, which serve different functions, protect and help people to cope with life. It's perfectly normal, for example, for more than one to be functioning at the same time. Generally, they only cause problems when two parts are in conflict and it prevents personal progress.

For instance, one part might be keen to promote a business, to go out and give talks while another doesn't want to stand up and be seen. Both parts, and their responses, are likely to have been established in childhood, but sometimes the messages get muddled and this can be seen in adulthood when a conflicting part pushes back, generally as a way of offering protection.

Connecting the parts

When this happens, it can be useful to explore what's going on and to try to discover why one part is discouraging or sabotaging the pursuit of heartfelt desires or bringing unhappiness. One way to do this and to find resolution is through parts therapy. Although historically it was employed mainly by hypnotherapists, for the past 30 years, ego-state therapy has been used by many psychotherapists. It has also been used by eye movement desensitisation and reprocessing (EMDR) practitioners – including psychologists, hypnotherapists, counsellors and psychotherapists – in the treatment of acute and chronic post-traumatic stress disorder.

With awareness, a felt sense and conflict-resolution skills, it can also be used as an independent tool for day-to-day inner resolutions. It's particularly effective where a person has already tried several approaches to overcome an issue, but they still feel at odds or conflicted. Learning how to identify and negotiate with our ego states can help to explain how personality is structured and provide an approach for lasting change. According to Gordon, it can also help with physical health and lead to an improved inner dialogue and a greater understanding of the self.

'Nobody can bring you peace but yourself'
Ralph Waldo Emerson

HOW TO IDENTIFY CHALLENGING PARTS

Grab a notepad or sheet of paper and make a list of situations that feel...

...conflicted
Perhaps you want to move to the countryside for more space and nature, but equally you really enjoy the social aspects and choice found in city living?

...ambivalent
Is there a part of you that would love to have kids and another part that really doesn't like the idea?

...confused
Are you keen to get a promotion at work, but something feels awry and you can't put your finger on what it is?

...stuck
Maybe both you and your partner want to get married, but you can't seem to progress things despite their willingness and enthusiasm?

....

....

....

....

....

....

....

...contradictory
Do you publicly profess to be a dedicated environmentalist, but never remember to put out the recycling?

....

....

....

....

....

....

....

Now, read back on what you've written. Does it provide any new or surprising insights? Are some situations repetitions of the same thing? Are two or more of your answers linked?

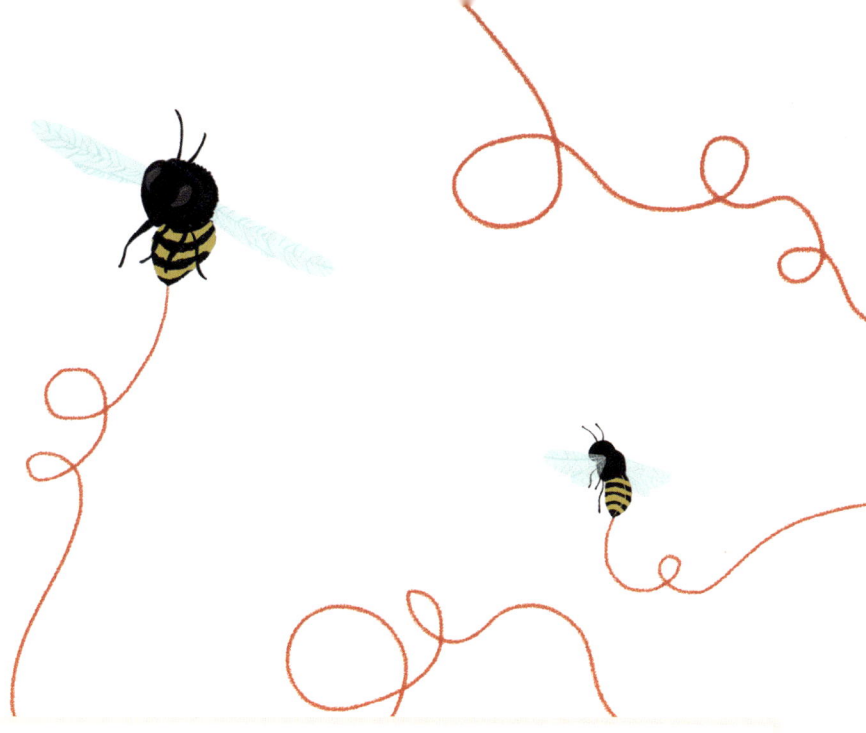

With this in mind...
...it's possible to view the parts more closely and work at ways to resolve any that are in conflict. Here's how:

- Identify both roles. You could refer to the two parts as 'conflicting' and 'motivating'. First, try to identify the latter, the one that is keen for action or change. Next, pinpoint the former, the part that is thwarting your preference or desire on a deeper level.

- Cultivate compassion. A motivating part might express itself with a lot of energy and sometimes aggression towards its conflicting counterpart. Keep in mind that both parts – and many others – make up you. They are there to help. Try to observe and regard them with acceptance and compassion.

- Work towards resolution. Once you have identified the conflicting parts you'd like to work with, think about giving them the opportunity to communicate and come to an agreement on how to work together. This can be done independently using dialoguing or self-hypnosis.

DIALOGUING

First, give each of the motivating and conflicting parts a name. For example, the former might be a desire to start a business, this feels full of hope and excitement – let's call it Skye. The latter is safer in the job it knows and might be wary of self-employment, let's call this Sam. You could write or draw a character sketch of both and label them with their respective emotions and attributes.

Now, take two or three minutes to tap into the feeling and sense you get from each part (eyes can be closed or open). Next, allow the two to converse for between two and 10 minutes, without stopping to ponder, edit or correct the script. Here's an example of how it might begin, but the idea is to chart your own conversation between the conflicting parts:

Skye: Hi, Sam, will you talk to me?
Sam: Okay, ask me a question or make a statement and I'll respond.
Skye: What is your job?
Sam: This feels really odd! Okay. I'm here to protect you in case something happens.
Skye: Thank you for protecting me. Can I ask, what are you worried about? What is it that you need?

....

....

....

....

....

....

....

....

....

....

....

....

It might feel as though you're making it up, and really, you are. Remember, however, that you have all the answers within. It's perfectly natural to feel self-conscious. Try to keep going with it, even if it seems a bit strange. The insights and details that emerge can be surprising.

SELF-HYPNOSIS

This might sound daunting, but it's more straightforward than often imagined. The main elements include your preferred method of relaxation, visualisation and self-guided prompts.

Here's one example:

1. Relax. In a quiet space, take a few deep breaths and close your eyes. Aim for five to 10 minutes of relaxation or mindfulness, using the breath as an anchor.

2. Feel. Gently, invite each part, one at a time, to rise. Tap into what you feel when each one stands up. From which part of the body does each part surface? What feeling does it embody – fearful, curious, angry, excited?

3. Name. Try to cultivate a strong sense of each part. You might like to attribute a colour, shape or name to identify its characteristics.

4. Communicate. Ask each part if it is happy to talk to you today. Wait for a felt response. This might be a feeling or a sense in your body or mind. Invite each one to speak to the other in turn and see what they have to say. Act as an intermediary. Encourage open dialogue.

5. Negotiate. Sometimes the conflicting part might not want to stand back. If that happens, you will need to negotiate. Always be patient and wait for at least a couple of minutes in between each question if need be.

6. Explain. If need be, tell the conflicting part that another area is unhappy and that improved communication between it and them might encourage harmony. Suggest that a few small ideas or tweaks could make both happier.

7. Summarise. Outline the role each plays. For example: 'Conflicting part, can you see how important it is for motivating part to deliver a confident presentation?' or 'Motivating part, can you see that conflicting part is trying to protect you?'

8. Resolve. Try to come to a resolution. Ask the conflicting part if it can work in unison with its motivating colleague. It's akin to trying to resolve an argument between friends.

9. Gratitude. Remember to thank each part for the work it's doing to protect you and help you grow.

10. Stay in touch. You might need to return at a later point to explore any unresolved areas. Remain diplomatic, friendly, compassionate and grateful.

Please note that hypnotherapy or self-hypnosis isn't for everyone. It's not recommended if you have psychosis or certain types of personality disorder. If you have any concerns, please visit your GP before attempting any self-hypnosis exercises. For more information, visit nationalhypnotherapysociety.org and psychotherapy.org.uk.

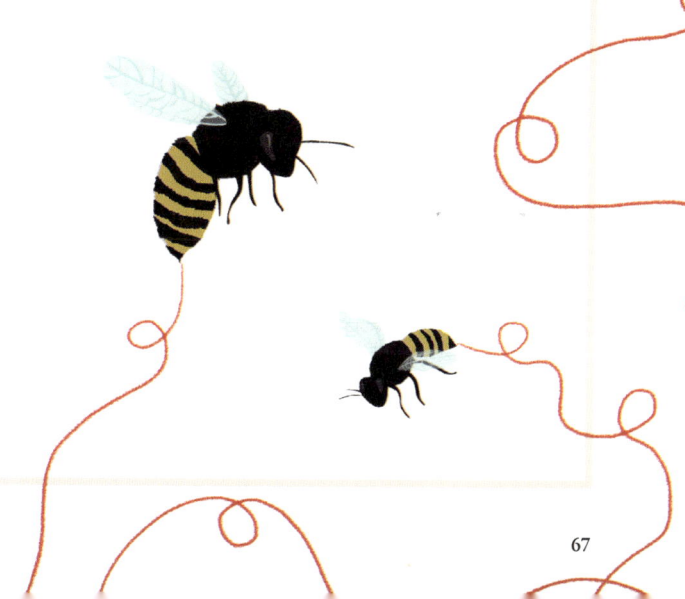

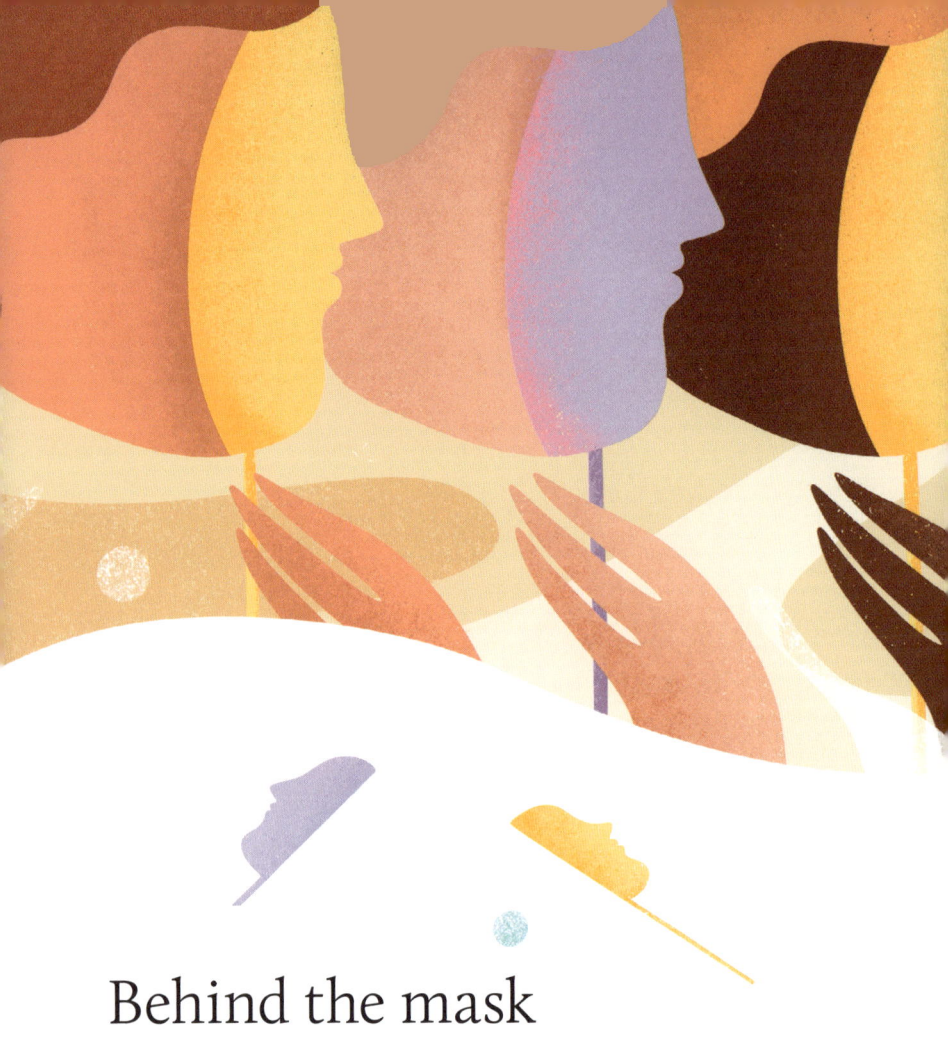

Behind the mask

Meditation provides an opportunity to cultivate awareness, drop any preconceived notions of who you are and tap into the true self. But what if your social camouflage is blocking the way?

Many animals use camouflage as a form of protection – polar bears' white coats help conceal them from other bears as well as poachers. Various types of lizard blend in with their surroundings to disguise themselves from predators. Humans also use a form of camouflage, not as a defence against physical dangers, but to shield themselves from social threat. Not being accepted, loved, nurtured or understood poses significant risks to wellbeing. From the moment a person is born, they adapt their behaviour to make sure they get the care they need. This social camouflage is known by psychologists as masking and is used to describe the process of blending in with the crowd.

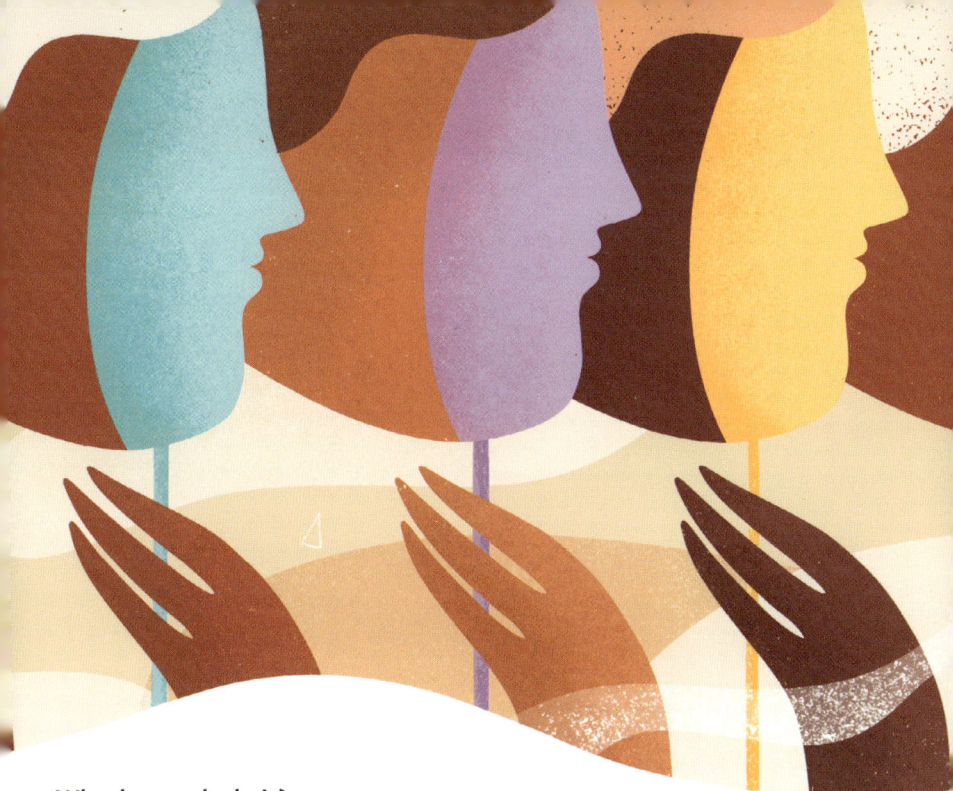

Why do people do it?

Fitting in with peers is a strategy inherited from primitive times. Being an outcast back then meant the chances of survival were dramatically reduced. These days, rather than simply ensuring physical safety, fitting in with other people contributes significantly to self-esteem.

Social media means that being liked and popular is seen as a measure of a person's worth more than ever before. Presenting a perfect version of your life is easy to do online. Some people will take 100 photos for every one that they post, and even then it'll be put through filters to make it even more appealing. But a form of editing happens offline, too – this is where social camouflage comes in. It might mean laughing at jokes that you don't find funny, pretending you enjoyed a book when you didn't, never going out without make-up or drinking more than you want to. Presenting yourself in a way that ensures you'll be liked and accepted is a growing pressure in the 21st century.

Everyone is different, and the pressure to conform to society's norms is felt unevenly. Some people are naturally shy, while others are more gregarious. Some learn in early childhood that being sociable is fun and positive, while others associate it with being criticised and vilified. Neurodiversity widens this spectrum still further. Those with autism or attention deficit hyperactivity disorder, for example, might find they function more effectively in calm, quiet conditions, and that they feel most relaxed on their own or in smaller groups. These differences, alongside social pressures, can exacerbate a sense that it's somehow necessary to hide who you really are.

Keeping up has a downside
Masking is an adaptive strategy to help ease social interactions, so it must be a good thing, right? Not entirely. While a little camouflaging can ease unfamiliar or awkward social situations, if you rely on it most of the time, it becomes a crutch. And if you don't feel comfortable being yourself, whether on social media or at a party, others won't get to know the real you.

When you doubt that you'll be accepted for your true self, or you feel unskilled socially, it's natural to think you need to change yourself to fit in. But while this might make you feel more secure, or even popular, it can be a false reward. Approval gained in this way can leave you wondering if it's the artificial version people want to be friends with rather than the genuine you, which can lead to anxiety and resentment. Constantly projecting an image of yourself that isn't authentic also takes energy and effort, so social events can be exhausting. Sometimes, keeping up a pretence can even leave you feeling disingenuous, which perpetuates a sense that who you really are isn't good enough.

Assessing the impact
Everyone uses social camouflage some of the time, but it can be helpful to pay attention to how much you rely on it to feel okay about yourself. To understand its place in your life, think about how you feel when you're attending social events, and then try asking yourself the following questions:

- Do you often make excuses to go to the bathroom so that you can relax and recharge for a moment?
- Do you feel exhausted after the event?
- Do you feel like you're playing a role?
- Do you lie about your views and your experiences?
- Do you crave being alone so that you can be your true self?
- Do you have to wear make-up when you're with others?

If most of your answers are 'yes', you might be using masking to the detriment of your authentic self.

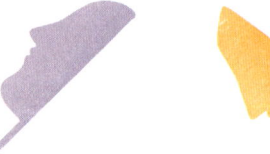
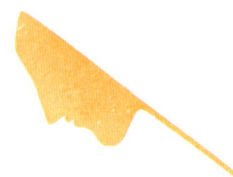

'Your time is limited, so don't waste it living someone else's life'
Steve Jobs

Breaking the cycle

Do you want others to know the true you so that you're liked for who you genuinely are? Saving social camouflage as a tool for those occasional unnerving social situations means that you can build up your confidence to be your authentic self in all other settings. Dropping your guard might mean you'll sometimes say or do something that others don't agree with or that doesn't receive everyone's approval. It could be that you find yourself standing alone now and then.

The risks might seem high, but the rewards are great. Knowing that you're liked for who you really are is a positive experience – and being loved by a few people for being the true you will lead to greater happiness than having a false version liked by many.

Dropping the disguise

This new way of being might make you feel more anxious in the short term. To help you through this transition you could try managing the anticipatory anxiety by playing energetic, uplifting music while getting ready, or repeating an affirming mantra before leaving the house, such as: 'I am free to be myself.' When you're back home, make your assessment of the event more productive by journalling or recording a voice note detailing all your feelings about it. Then recuperate with a cosy drink, a hot bath or a cosy pair of PJs.

Over time, seeing when it's necessary to camouflage and when it isn't will come more naturally. Your self-esteem and confidence will grow as you realise that people still want to spend time with you no matter how shy, eccentric or otherwise authentic you are. Social camouflage is a natural and inevitable part of life, but using it as an optional tool rather than an essential crutch means you have ultimate control.

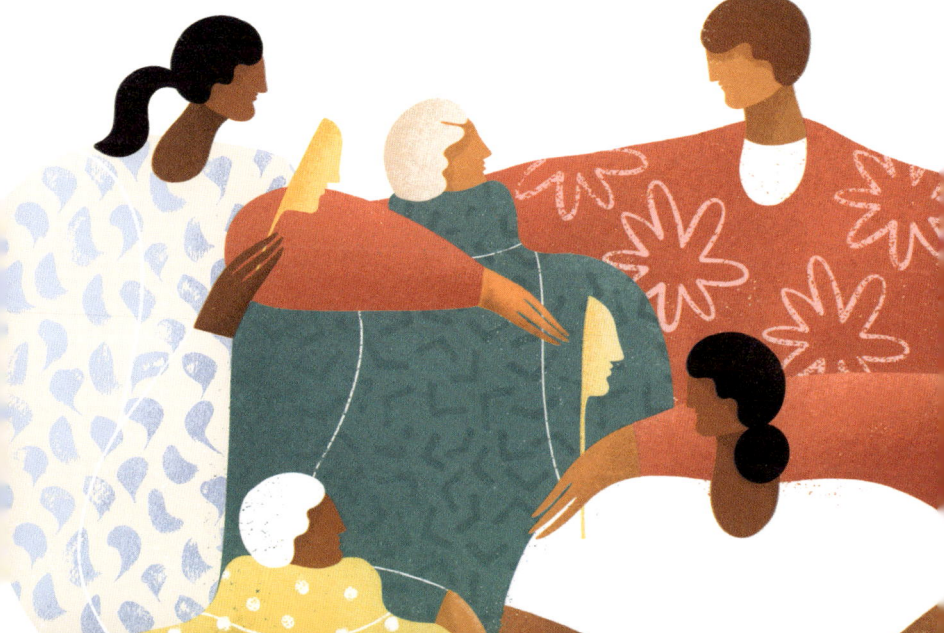

HOW TO BE YOUR TRUE SELF

If you feel ready to begin to break cover, here are some tips on how to do it, small step by small step:

1. Identify the person with whom you feel most comfortable in a social situation and start by being a bit more natural with them. Open up to them about your worries about not being your true self and ask if they could bear with you while you peel away the protective layers. If it feels okay, you could also ask them for feedback about how you're doing. Use the space below to note what they say.

2. Once you've built up your confidence with this person, try being your authentic self with someone in whose company you feel a little less comfortable. Work your way through different people and social situations, slowly building up to the most anxiety-provoking situation of all – whether that's a room full of unfamiliar people in a new setting or an old group of friends with whom you've been trying to fit in. List possible people and situations here, from those that would make you feel least anxious to most.

3. You might feel vulnerable without your usual armour in place, so prepare by building up your inner social coach. Talk to yourself in a positive, encouraging way. If you find this difficult to do, imagine yourself as a child going into the situation – what would you say to encourage and support the younger version of you?

4. Most communication is non-verbal. At home, practise standing tall and looking up and out. Rehearse slow, deep breathing to calm your body and mind. Use these techniques when you're out and about. Have you ever noticed that someone else is anxious in your presence? What would you say to them to calm them?

REAL TALK

Use the three columns below to help organise your thoughts about when you use masking and to brainstorm ways you could introduce more authenticity.

Who I'm with...

....

....

....

....

....

....

....

What social camouflage am I using?
(For example, changing my voice, copying others' body language, concealing my real views.)

....

....

....

....

....

....

....

....

What can I do instead?
(For example, make sure I sit alongside someone I feel comfortable with, focus on being in my own body, be kind and honest about my opinion.)

> 'Only from the heart can you touch the sky'
>
> Rumi

Into the blue

How looking up can help to manage stormy thoughts on the ground

Have you ever lain on the grass and watched the sky on a summer's day? Perhaps it was vibrant blue and completely clear. Or maybe a few fluffy clouds were rolling by and peaceful birds were going about their business. As well as being relaxing to watch, the sky is a powerful metaphor that is widely used in meditation practices.

In Buddhist tradition, the sky evokes openness and freedom. A central concept in Buddhism is Śūnyatā, which translates as 'emptiness' or 'voidness'. It refers to the absence of anything solid and enduring. In his book, *Sacred Tibet*, artist, teacher and author Philip Rawson notes that in Tibetan Buddhist art 'one potent metaphor for the Void... is the sky'. It's an empty and infinite backdrop to the ever-changing weather. Buddhism teaches that everything, including the contents of the mind, appears and disappears naturally. Śūnyatā is seen as a freeing and blissful state, often achieved in meditation by appreciating this transient quality.

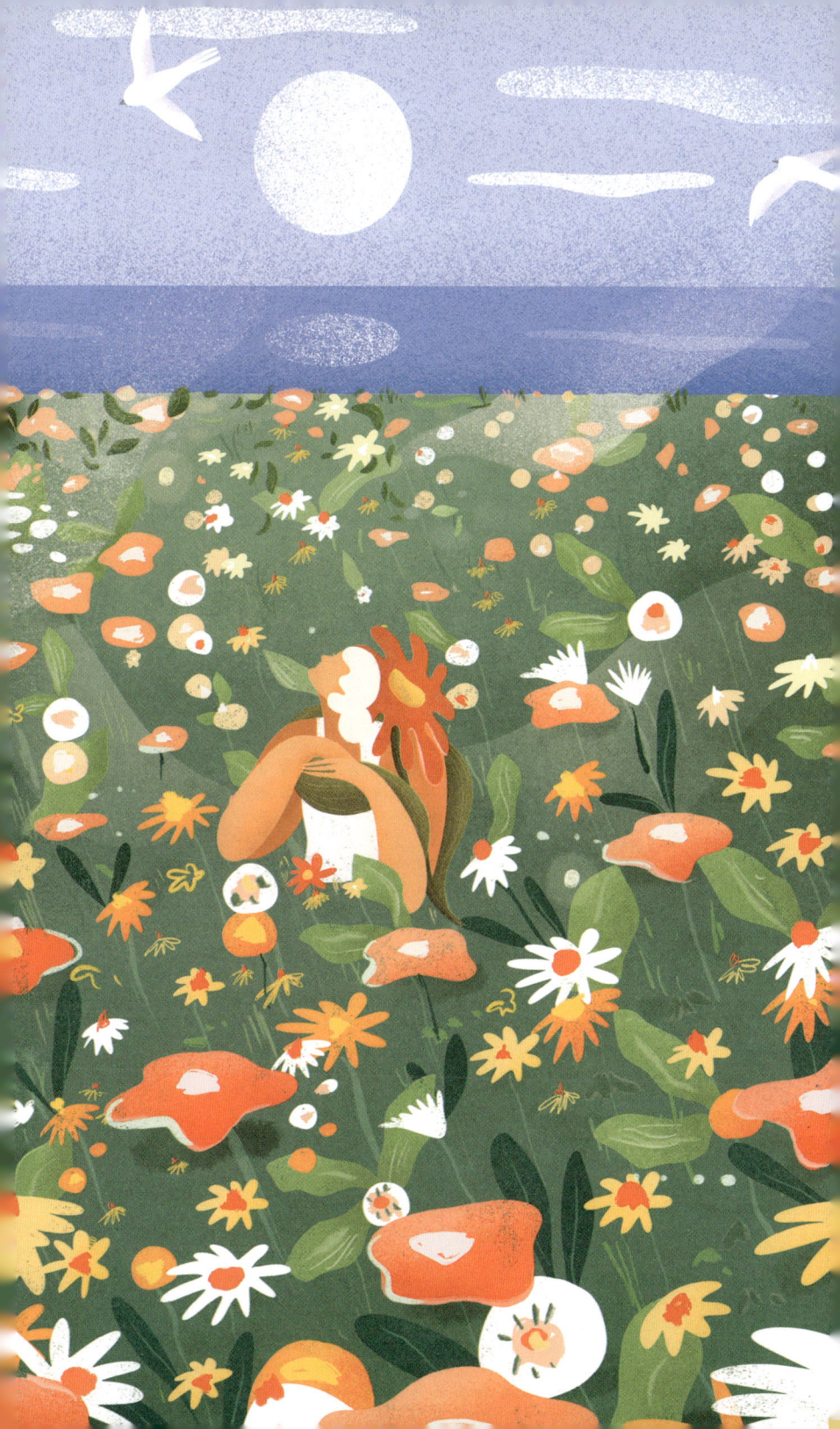

Western interpretation

Western mindfulness, which has its roots in Buddhist tradition, frequently turns to the sky analogy. Within this, the practitioner is fully in the moment, observing thoughts and feelings without judging them. They're given space to drift through, like watching the weather without trying to control it. Even mindfulness-based therapies, such as Acceptance and Commitment Therapy (ACT), draw on the calming image of the sky. ACT guides people to manage their thoughts using a technique called cognitive defusion, where they are encouraged to separate themselves from any distressing beliefs and to then reframe them to reduce their power.

In a similar way, the blue-sky metaphor can be used in meditation practice, so that rather than suppressing challenging thoughts and difficult emotions, the practitioner allows them to become clouds that are accepted before they gradually dissipate. When doing this, it can help to use the following key to delve deeper into the metaphor:

Remember the blue sky

Author and Headspace co-founder Andy Puddicombe says: 'Clouds come and go. We tend to get caught up in the clouds and forget about the blue sky.' Meditation is about reconnecting to the underlying stillness of the mind that, like the sky, is a constant backdrop to the changing conditions.

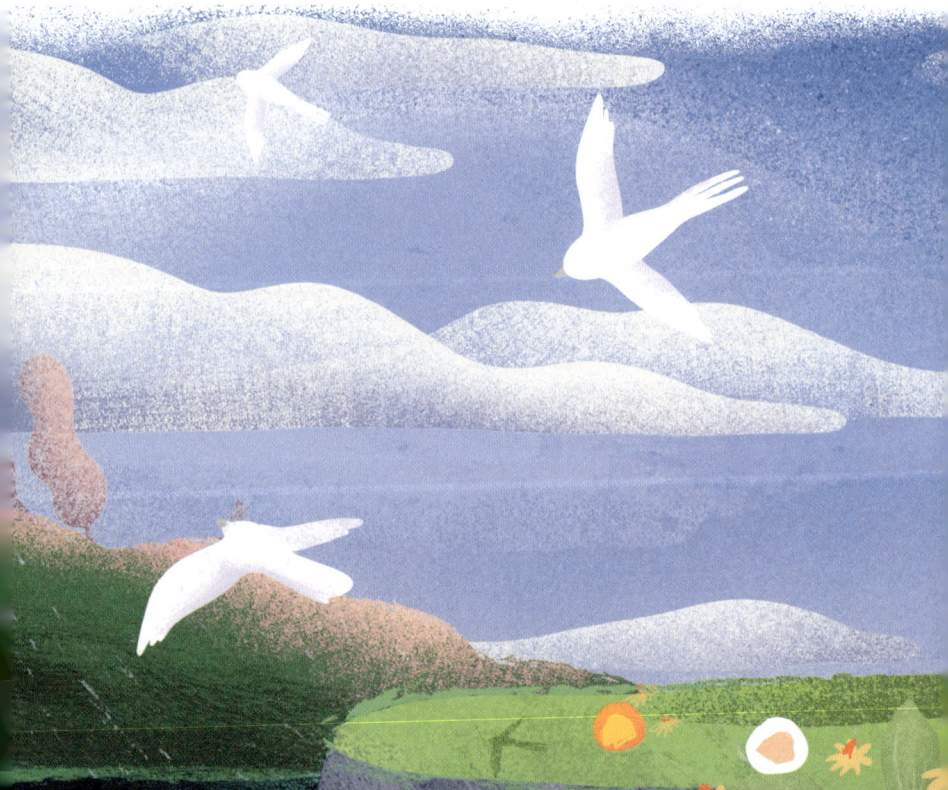

Watch the weather

Blue sky isn't contrived, but a part of nature. Similarly, meditation isn't about trying to do or change anything. It's pausing and noticing what's happening in the mind. Thoughts and feelings can't be stopped in their tracks, just as clouds can't be grasped, shaped or erased. Sit and watch them go by.

Let the storms pass

Sometimes, the mind is calm and clear, like a bright summer's day, on other occasions it's volatile and cloudy. The metaphor is a reminder that even when it's hidden behind life's stormy moments, a bright, blue sky is waiting to return.

A challenging mood can be thought of as dark, heavy fog, or a particular anxiety can be envisioned as a large, looming rain cloud that demands attention. It might feel like the whole sky is grey, but even when the weather's inclement, remember that up above the clouds, the blue remains. In meditation, you can go above the clouds and rest there. As Zen master and author Thich Nhat Hanh said: 'Even if it is very foggy, cloudy or stormy, the blue sky is always there, for us, above the clouds.'

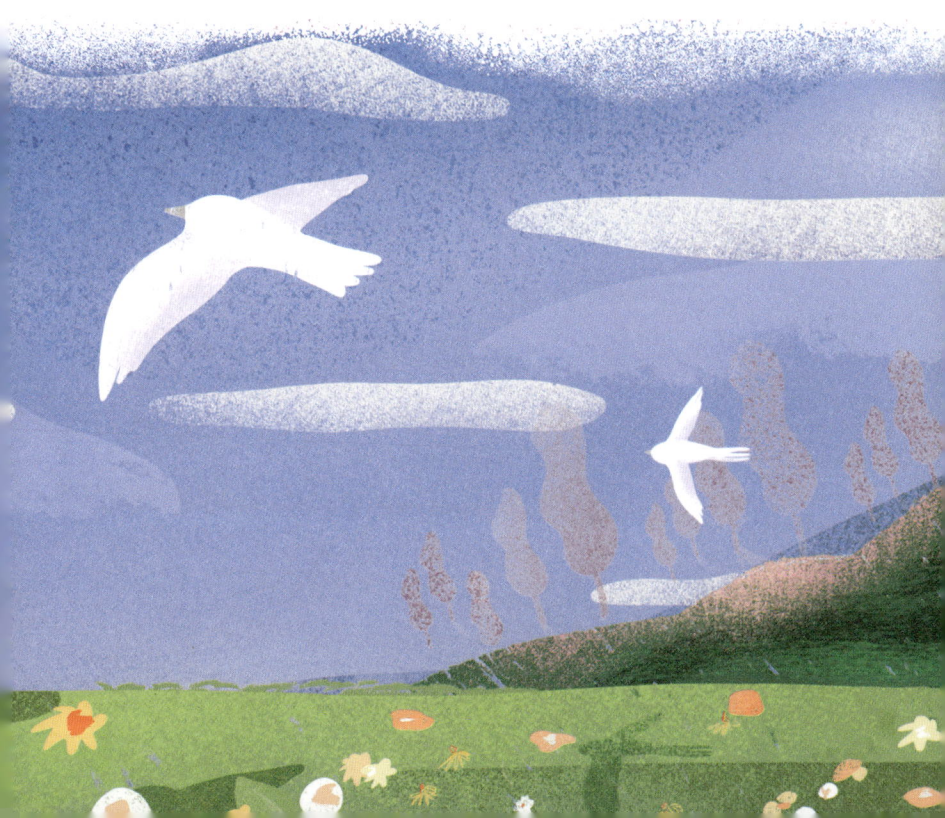

BLUE-SKY STATE OF MIND MEDITATION

Christoph Spiessens is a certified mindfulness teacher, author and founder of the Manchester Mindfulness Festival. In this guided meditation, the image of the blue sky is used as a point of focus to create a sense of calmness and clarity.

1. Find a safe and comfortable space. You can do this brief meditation either sitting or lying down. Close your eyes if that feels okay. Alternatively, lower your gaze or focus softly on an object such as a plant or a tree outside your window. Adopt a posture that embodies a sense of wakefulness and take a few deep, conscious breaths.

2. As best you can, bring to mind a blue sky with clouds of various sizes. See them drifting by. Your mind will naturally wander when you meditate. This is entirely normal. Thoughts come and go all the time, just like the clouds. Being in the observer seat, notice how your thoughts pop up, float by and then disappear. Experiment with observing them without being consumed by them. You can try to broadly label the thought clouds, such as work, social, family, for example. This involves parts of the cognitive brain that can downregulate the emotional brain.

3. Consider how the practice made you feel. Do you perhaps notice a renewed sense of space between you and your thoughts?

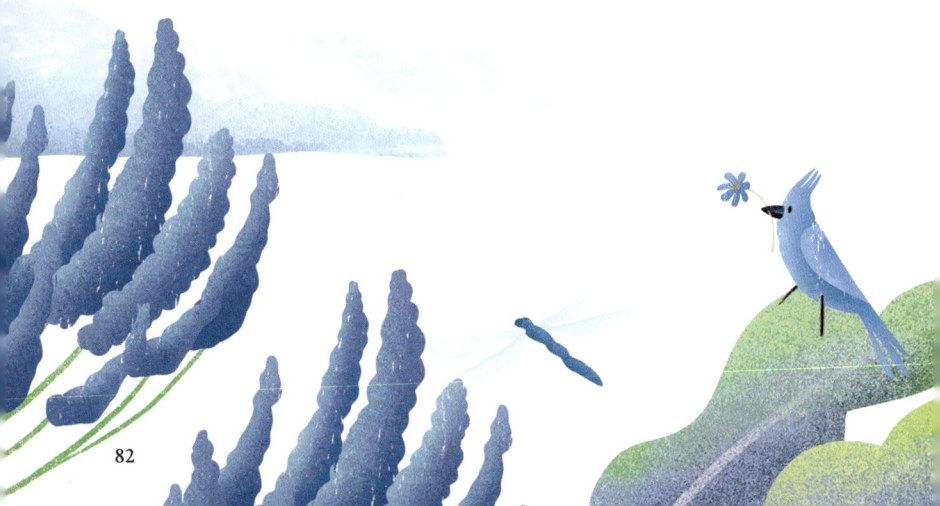

CHOOSE YOUR METAPHOR

There are lots of different analogies that can be used to observe thoughts and feelings. If you're struggling to picture a blue sky, try another image. Here are a few you could consider:

A train station
You're on the platform and your thoughts are the trains pulling in. Rather than climbing aboard every single one, you stand back and watch them depart the station in turn.

A cinema
Picture yourself at the movies with the contents of your mind being played on the big screen. While you might be engrossed in the unfolding scenes, you're aware that there's a distance between you and the screen, and that the film will eventually end.

A river
Water constantly flows over a riverbed. In the same way, thoughts, feelings and experiences always flow through the mind. Imagine your mind as a calm and constant free-flowing stream.

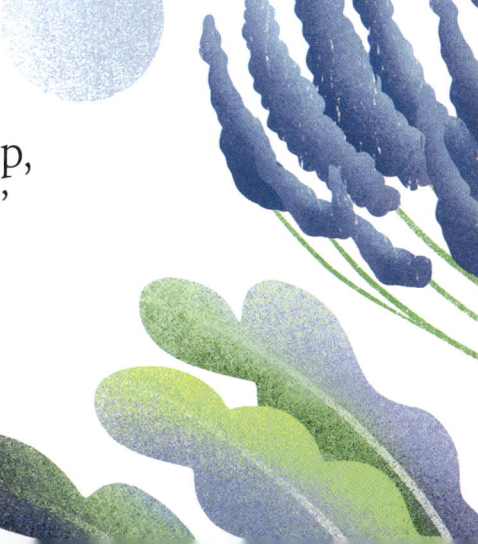

'Ah, but a man's reach should exceed his grasp, or what's a heaven for?'

Robert Browning

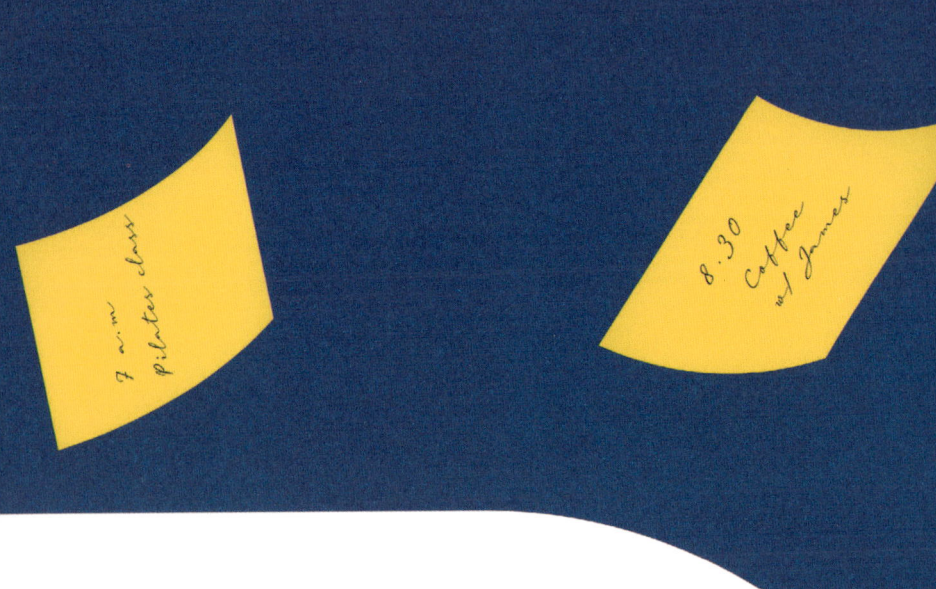

'Nature does not hurry,
yet everything is accomplished'

Lao Tzu

Swerve from your path

Focus is sometimes overrated. To live a full life, it's also necessary to step into the pleasure and power of distraction

If you ever feel like you spend too much of your life rushing around, ticking things off to-do lists, perpetually racing to get to the next appointment, thinking ahead and planning where you've got to go next, you're not alone.

But have you ever stopped to wonder what you're missing when you move through your day in this fast-paced, productive-yet-never-enough approach to time that leaves you blinkered and unable to fully witness the world around you? *New York Times* bestselling author, speaker and poet Mark Nepo refers to this state in his essay, *Inside the Miracle*, when he says that succumbing to speed is a 'form of isolation'.

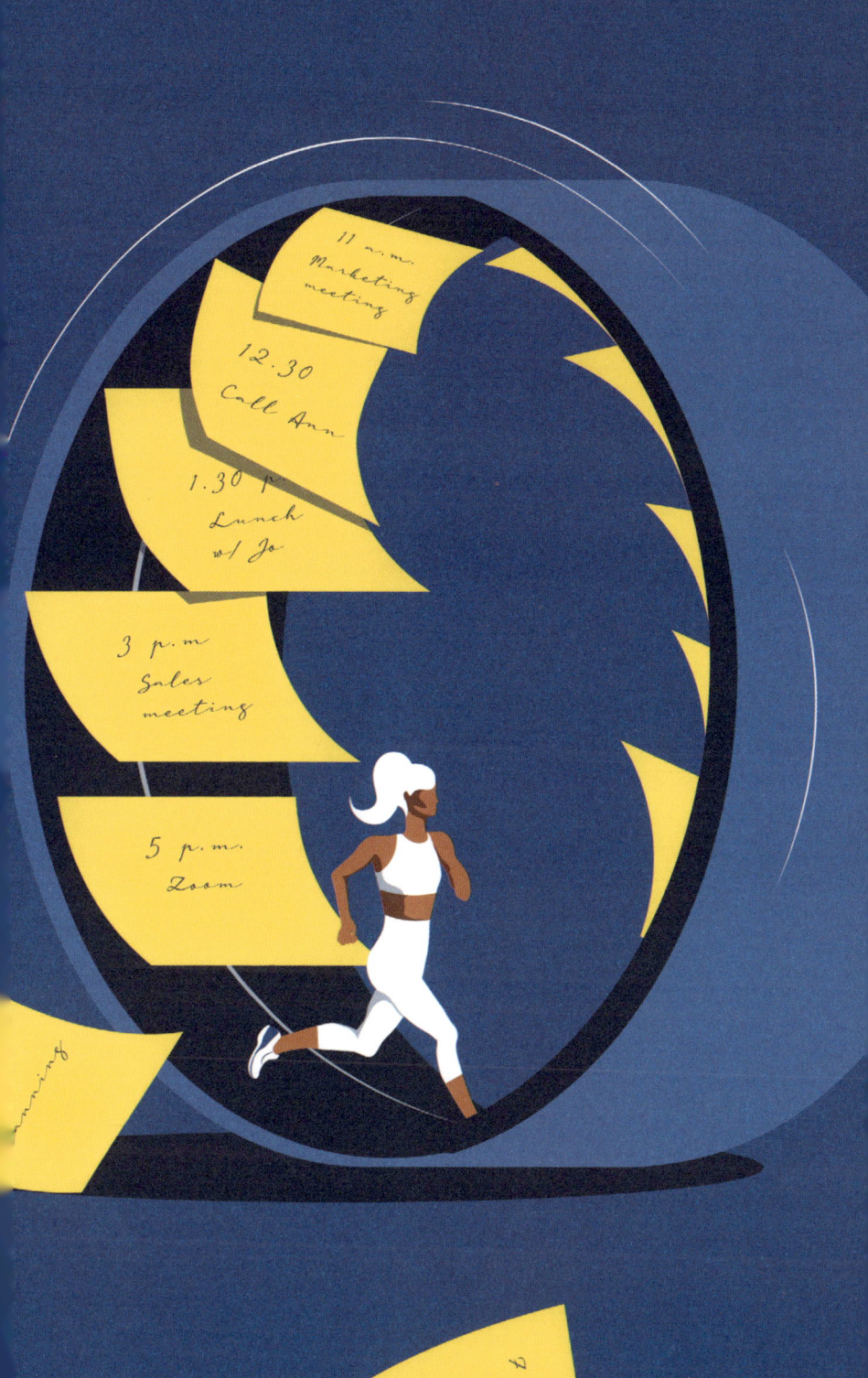

Dare to stray

But what if there was a different way of being? A way that encouraged kindness and connection along the way, while still honouring your commitments? What if, once in a while, you allowed yourself to swerve from your path? Author, Buddhist teacher and psychologist Tara Brach discusses this concept in her book, *Trusting the Gold*, and highlights three points:

- 'Swerving from our scheduled paths is not something we easily do.'
- 'Focusing on our own concerns and stress can put us in a trance, covering over our natural sensitivity and compassion.'
- 'And by managing life from our mental control towers, we have separated ourselves from our bodies and hearts.'

By pausing – even when in a rush – and noticing what's going on around you, rather than reacting out of frustration and anger, it's possible both to avoid conflict and improve quality of life.

This is exactly what UCLA professor and author Cassie Mogilner discovered in a study she led at the University of Pennsylvania in the US. In an experiment where subjects were assigned a range of different tasks, those who paused to notice others' needs and stop what they were doing to help ended up feeling as though they had more time, not less. In an interview with the *Harvard Business Review*, Cassie explains: 'People who give time feel more capable, confident and useful. They feel they've accomplished something and, therefore, that they can accomplish more in the future. And this self-efficacy makes them feel that time is more expansive.'

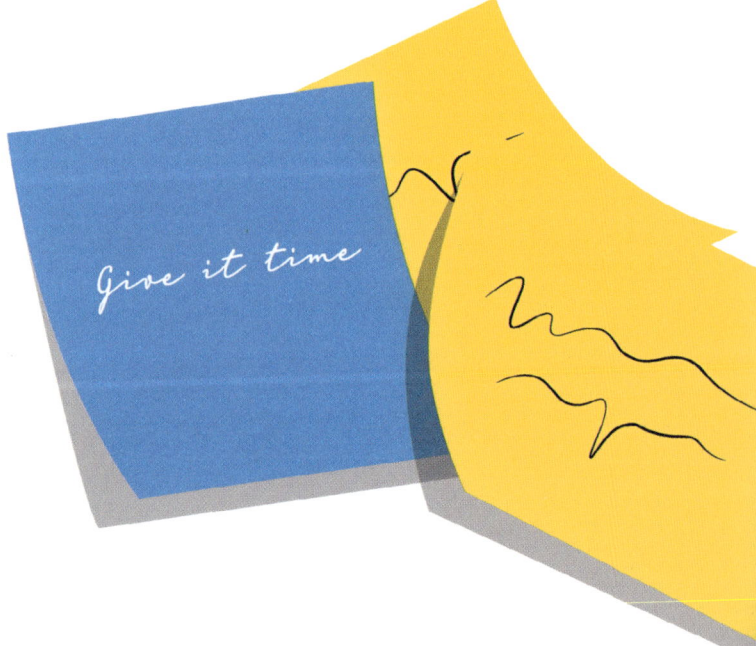

Negative tendencies

But if this benevolent approach to the world is so beneficial, why don't more people adopt it more often? The truth is, it's hard and goes against fear-based instincts. When under pressure, people are more likely to adopt a negativity bias. Making a conscious effort to slow down – even if it's just the breath – when in a rush, and using the imagination to see the good in those who appear to be in the way, takes practice.

This is something that self-development coach and author Roxie Nafousi refers to in her book, *Manifest*, where she explains that people have around 60,000 repetitive thoughts a day. Of those, approximately 80 per cent are negative: 'To begin to undo repetitive, negative and limiting ways of thinking, we must commit to consistent practice and repeatedly choose to nourish our mind by replacing negative thoughts with empowering ones,' she says.

So, when you're in a queue at the supermarket checkout or stuck behind a chronically slow driver and you hear your inner voice saying things like: 'This person is getting in my way,' hit pause. Then try to replace the thought with: 'Who knows what might be going on in this person's life right now?' And use your imagination to conjure up a range of challenging experiences, from illness to relationship difficulties, that they might be dealing with. Because the truth is, you don't know.

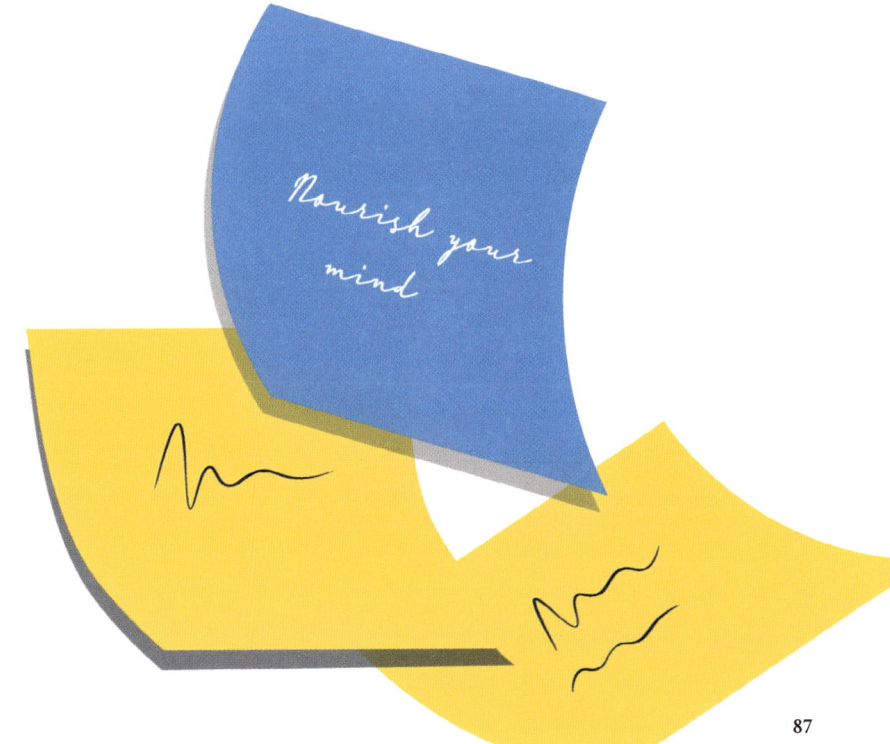

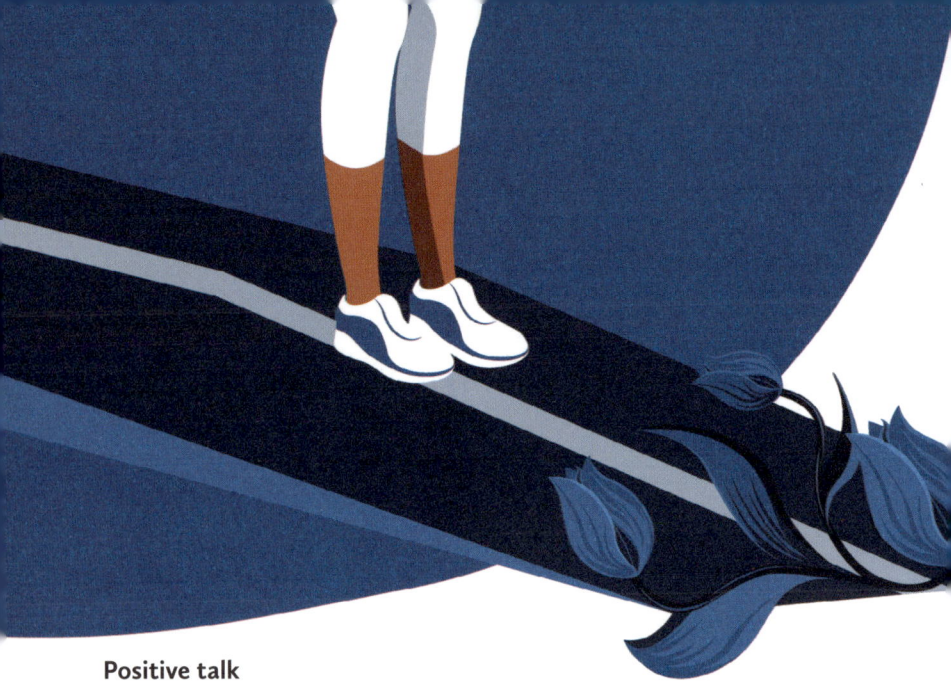

Positive talk

Likewise, the thought: 'I'm going to be late and my day will be ruined,' is likely to speed up your breathing and get your heart racing, sending you into a state of near panic. Rather than succumbing to the fear, try gently telling yourself: 'Everything will be okay and things will work out exactly as they should.' It's amazing how powerful and soothing it feels to offer yourself compassion by changing your inner dialogue. 'Instead of imagining the worst possible outcome, imagine the best,' Roxi suggests.

According to psychologist Karen Kwong repeatedly replacing negative thoughts with positive ones can even change the brain. 'Essentially, the brain can reorganise pathways, create new connections, and possibly even new neurons, at any stage in life, because of what we've learned,' she says.

This is fortuitous, given that straying, or allowing ourselves to get distracted, isn't often seen as the best approach when it comes to the health and plasticity of our brains. 'While it's true that staying focused on the task at hand encourages plasticity and increases longevity, certain kinds of distraction can also be a good thing,' adds Karen. 'Focus and flexibility are equally important. If you want to lead a purposeful life, it is likely to come with all sorts of twists and turns. That's why I always advise my clients to follow their curiosity, even if it means straying from the path they've set out for themselves.

'To use a military acronym, we live in a VUCA world (volatile, uncertain, complex and ambiguous) and the individuals and businesses who came out the least scathed by the pandemic were those who had a strong sense of purpose and clear values, while being able to adapt to the ever-changing environment.

'It's easy to get fooled into thinking that life is a straight line and once we've chosen our course, whether that's pursuing a particular career or sticking to a schedule we've set out for the day, we have to stick with it. But that's not true.'

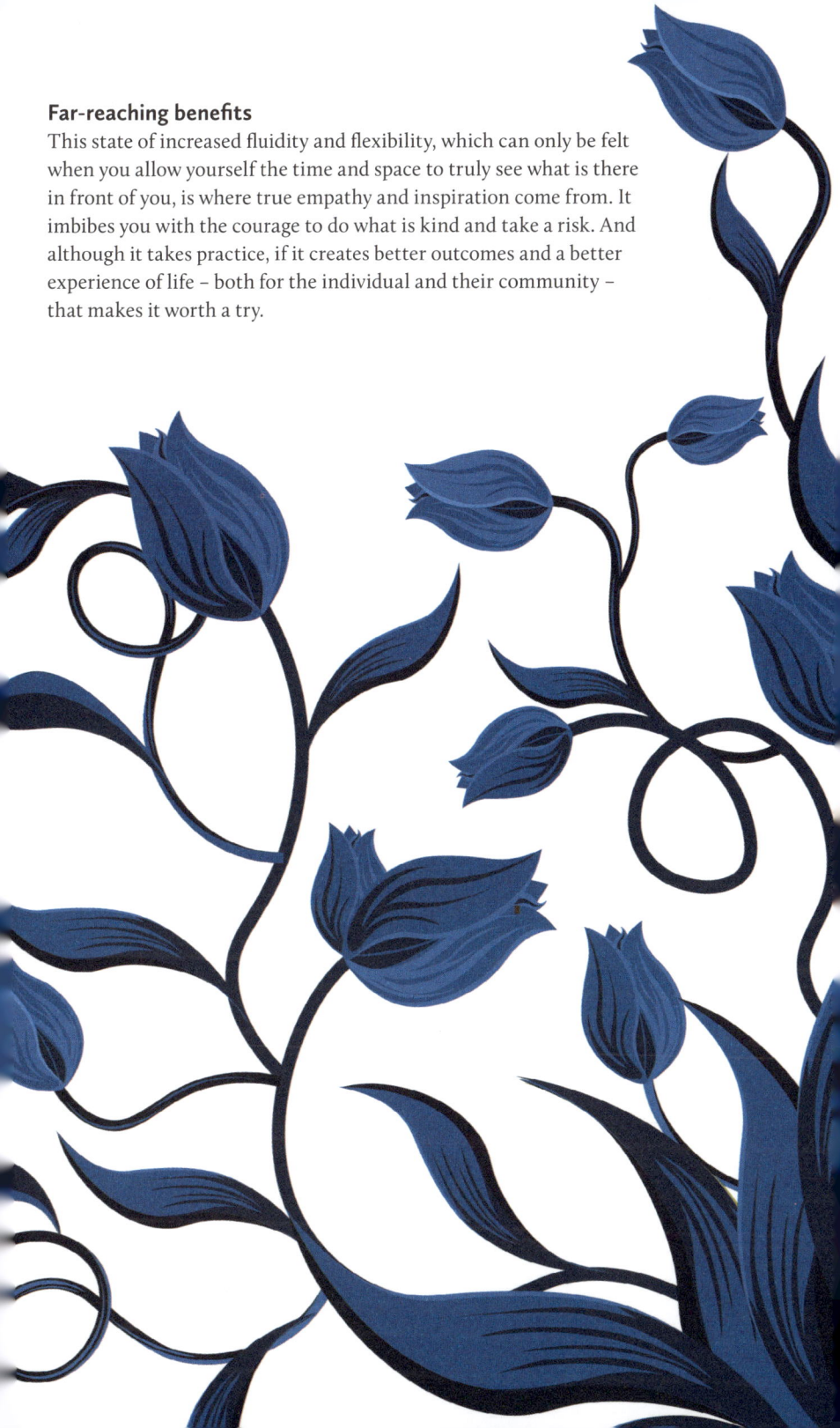

Far-reaching benefits
This state of increased fluidity and flexibility, which can only be felt when you allow yourself the time and space to truly see what is there in front of you, is where true empathy and inspiration come from. It imbibes you with the courage to do what is kind and take a risk. And although it takes practice, if it creates better outcomes and a better experience of life – both for the individual and their community – that makes it worth a try.

VENTURE INTO THE UNKNOWN

Ways to feel more comfortable taking a different route.

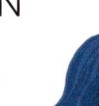

1. Journal on the idea of the unreal other
There's a sense that in an effort to prove and defend the self we become separate from each other. The truth is that most people have busy and difficult lives. Picture a person you saw as an obstruction recently. Perhaps it was a shop assistant you felt was going too slowly, or someone you dealt with on the phone with whom you were impatient. Try to imagine that person's life – their family and friends. Allow yourself to dwell on a range of different challenging situations that they might be struggling with at the moment.

....

....

....

....

....

....

....

....

....

....

....

2. Create a kindness meditation practice
Make room each day for two or three minutes where you see yourself in your mind's eye being kind to the people around you.

'At the end of a morning meditation, say out loud: "Please may I be kind,"' suggests Tara. 'Run through who you're going to be in touch with that day and spend a moment imagining a kind interaction between you so that you can stay attuned to kindness when you're with them.'

3. Develop mantras
'Whenever I repeat a mantra out loud or inside my head, I instantly feel more centred and empowered,' says Roxi. She claims mantras are a powerful way to increase empathy for others and help change your relationship with time. Choose a couple of phrases that resonate with you and repeat them in the morning, in moments throughout the day, such as when driving, and before bed.

You could try:
'I am calm, flexible and responsive to other people.'

'There is no need to rush, things usually work out exactly as they're supposed to.'

4. Plan distraction walks
These intentional rambles, where you allow yourself to take in your surroundings and be curious, work in both rural and urban environments. Go out with the aim of noticing at least five new things that you've previously overlooked, be they tiny insects, leaf shapes, unusual buildings or painted doorways. It'll help build up your sense that the world is a magical place where things are constantly unfolding outside of your direct experience. Record your thoughts here.

....

....

....

....

....

....

....

....

....

....

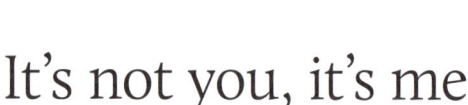

It's not you, it's me

Projection is a normal mental process where people attribute their own thoughts and feelings onto others – something that, in the world of social media, gets a little more complicated

Do you ever question what lies beyond the smokescreen of social media? When scrolling through feeds it can be interesting to notice whether the emotions that posts trigger in you are a response to other people or to a hidden part of yourself. The impact of social media on mental health is well documented and although digital platforms offer a beneficial place to communicate, express creativity and discover new things, sometimes the arena can lead to negative self-comparison, fuel a fear of missing out or leave you asking: 'Where am I in all of this?'

Digital diversion
Depending on how consciously you engage with social media, there might be times when online interactions result in a drop in energy, a sense of unease, irritation or even anxiety. Setting boundaries by deciding when and how to connect can be helpful. It can also be useful to build a clear understanding of what happens psychologically in the digital sphere, so you can protect yourself from the worst of its impact. One common psychological defence mechanism that you might experience in interactions with others is projection – it's a natural phenomenon that has its uses, but it can sometimes lead to misunderstandings and confusion.

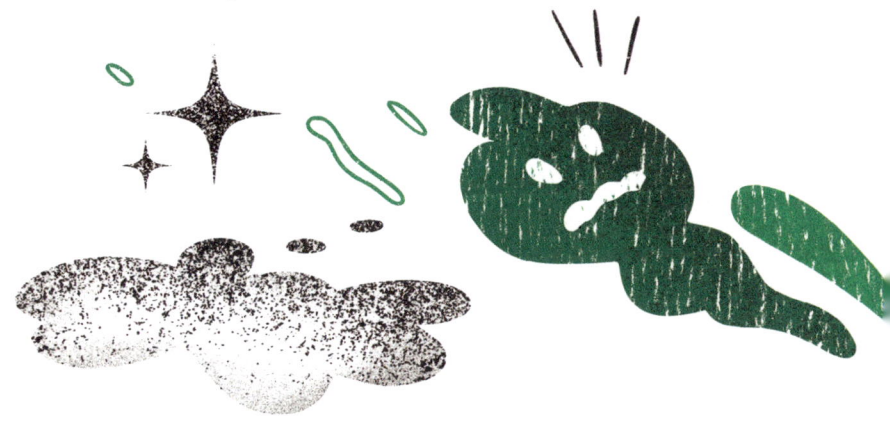

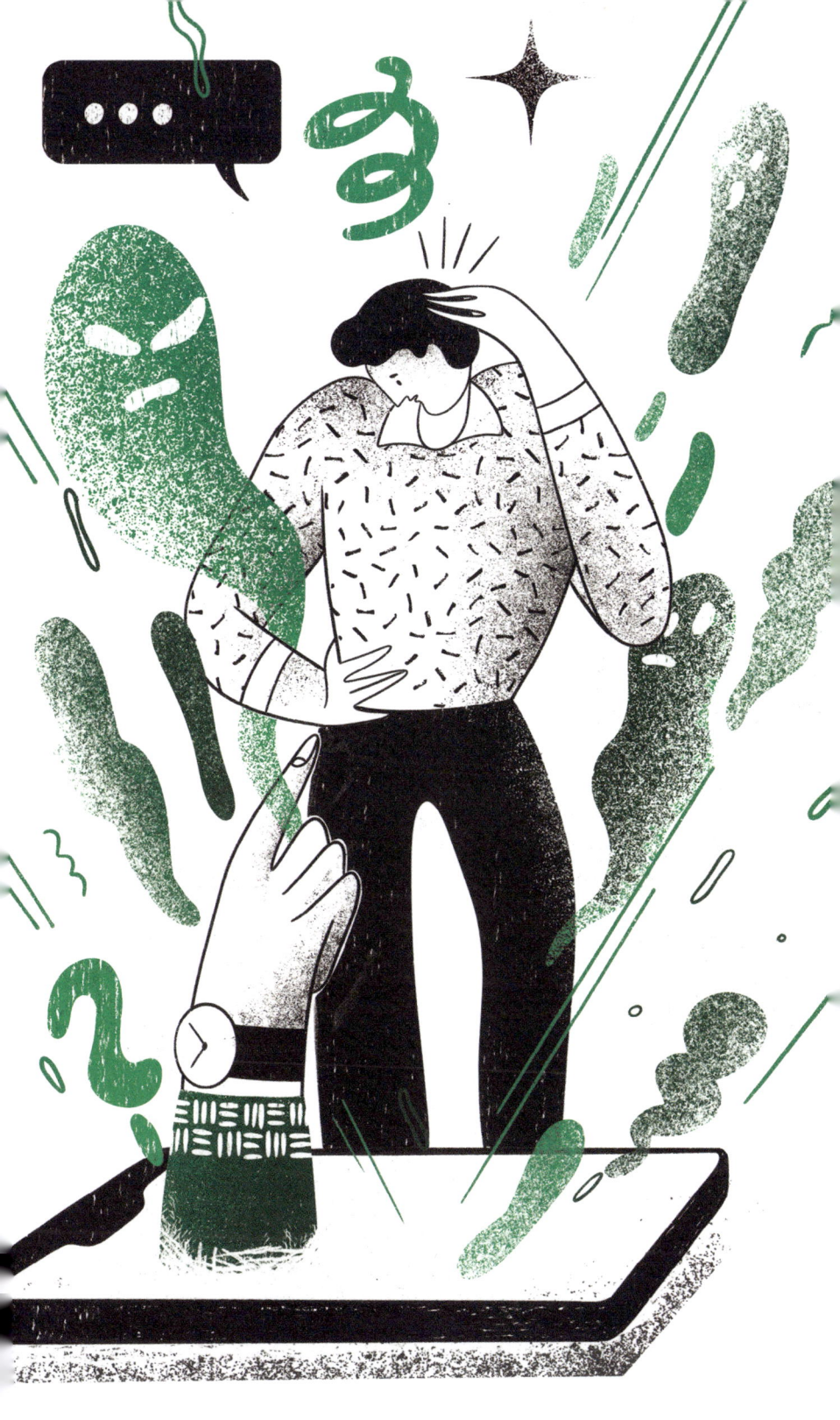

In the shadows

Projection is when you disown an aspect of your personality that isn't compatible with what you accept to be true about yourself; you project it (out of your awareness) onto another person and believe that this feeling or behaviour is coming from the other person instead. If, for example, a friend comments that a mutual acquaintance 'is being a bit careless' and adds 'I'm never that slapdash' it might be because there is a side of them that can be hurried and less considered at times. They've pushed this fact so far from their consciousness, however, that they just can't see it or admit it to themselves.

Although projection commonly occurs face-to-face, it also happens while scrolling on social media. Perhaps you've noticed this in your own interactions. You might project your conscious or unconscious thoughts and judgments onto others without realising it, leading you to believe the source of anxiety or irritation is coming from someone else. But the person might not be sending out the message you've received at all. It could be that their post has simply triggered an aspect of yourself about which you're in denial.

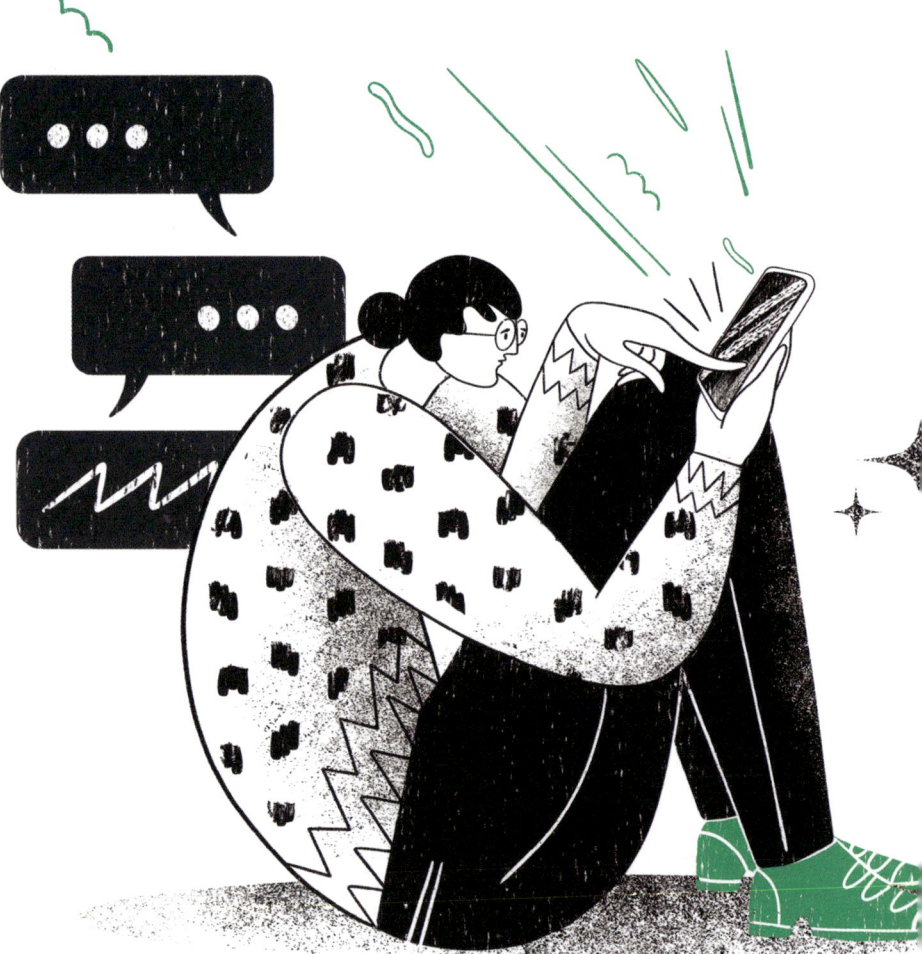

Hall of mirrors

UK psychotherapist Dave Mann likens projection to putting up a transparent projector screen between you and the other person. You can see this other person through the screen while simultaneously projecting a hologram of yourself onto that same space. You then interact with the other person as though you can see through both the screen and your own holographic image at the same time. The same layering can happen for the person on the other side, too.

Psychotherapist Nicole Jacob says: 'Projection is a natural, inevitable and necessary part of the human mind. We fill in the blanks and make assumptions about our environment and other people in order to live and make choices in the world. When we have to make a quick decision based on limited data, we're more likely to make mistakes, for example seeing a piece of fluff and thinking it's a spider. It costs us nothing to act as if the risk is real, so in that moment our brain responds as it would have done had it been a spider and flicks the fluff away. The imagined spider is as real to our brain as an actual spider.'

Nicole explains that in the digital realm it's possible to live in this projective state for extended periods of time. 'It's a wide space that you can project yourself into and [where you can] meet other projections. Sometimes, people may present more solid and real versions of themselves and sometimes we meet these "phantoms", deliberately created to pique and capture our attention. They arrive on our screens, but it is in our minds where the transformation happens, where we turn them into flesh and blood, which we then respond to as if they were real. It is this mental process that we can learn to become aware of and [thereby] regain a sense of control.'

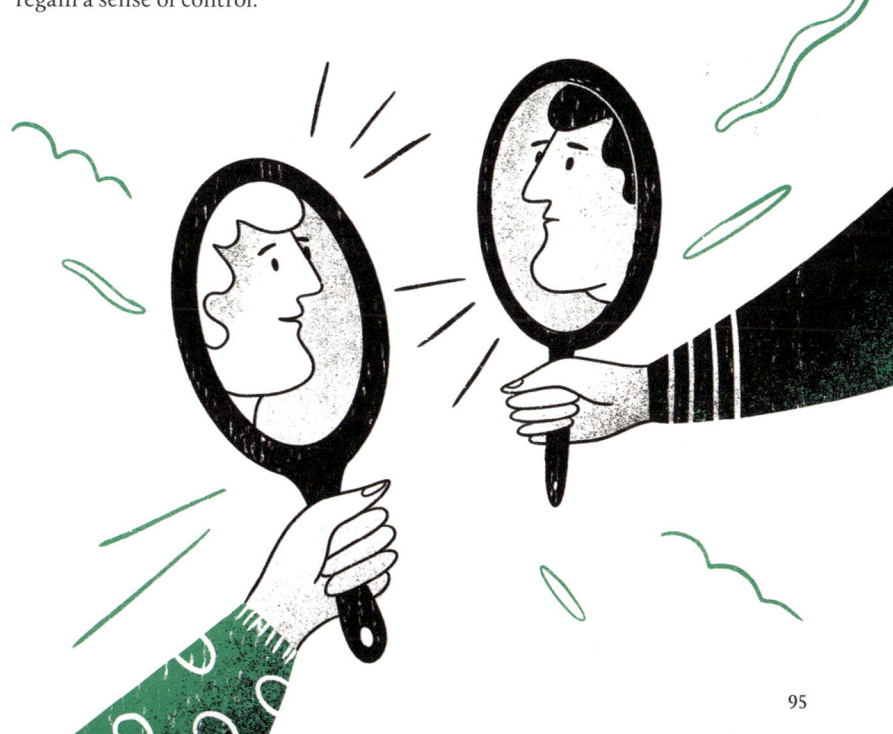

Shades of grey

So projection is when you attribute a personal quality, trait or attitude that you've disowned onto the post you're reading or account you're viewing. For example, say you're following someone and you think something along the lines of 'Goodness, they seem to be showing off a bit here'. It may be that they're being boastful. But there's also a chance they're not. It could be you've disowned a similar quality, such as a capacity for having visibility, a voice or being proud of your talents.

Conversely, you might follow an expert in a particular field whom you consider to be brilliant. If you seem to put them on a pedestal, it could be that you are disowning your own brilliance. Either way, it isn't always easy to notice your own thought process and whether you're projecting. There are various factors at play in the situation at any given time. Understanding projection, therefore, isn't always clear-cut.

'It's safe to say that whether it's an in-person interaction or one on social media, it can be tricky to sometimes identify whether we are experiencing a projection or not,' says Nicole. '[With the latter,] in the absence of being able to check with the real world, it can feel as though what we are seeing or being told is true. There are a lot of blanks on social media – we're not given the whole story, and even when we are shown an accurate portrayal, we don't always see the full picture. This happens in real life, too. So, often, we fill in the information that is missing with material from our own patterns and insights.'

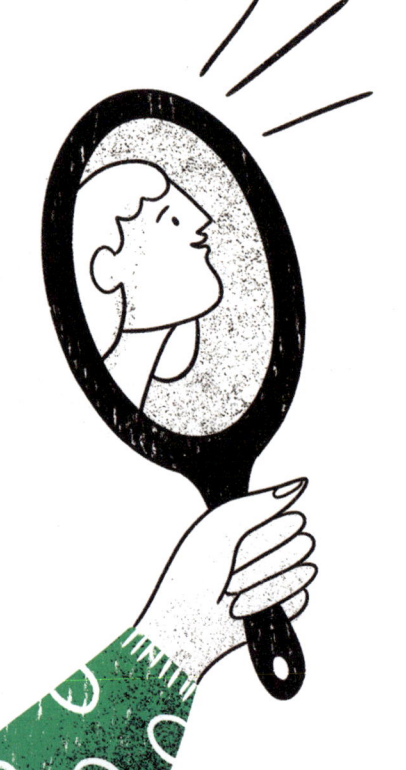
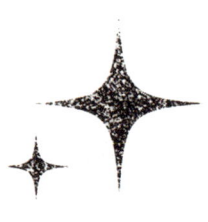

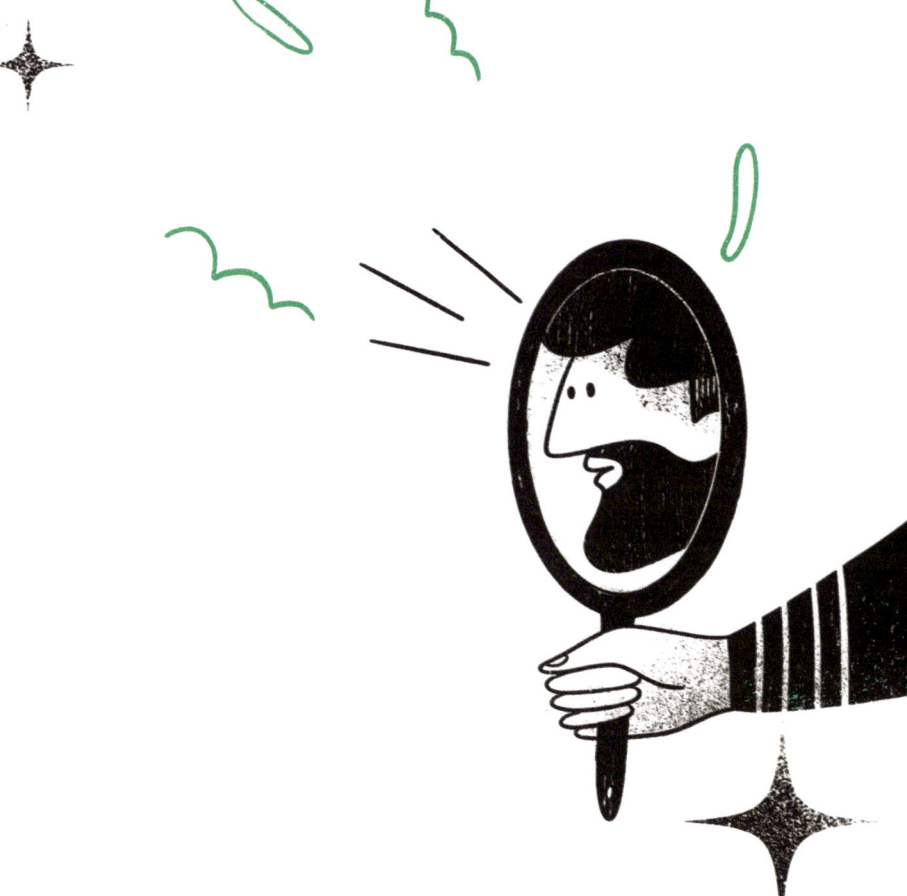

Raising awareness

There are times when projection can be helpful. Some might post an item or even start a social media account as a way to play with how they present themselves to the world. Perhaps they might be consciously showing themselves as they truly are or maybe they're experimenting with another version of themselves – how they wish they were or how they might be if certain things were different. This is a way to explore identity.

Noticing your patterns and starting to understand what belongs to you is an important first step. Having an awareness of your patterns, thoughts and feelings can be helpful in adopting a mindful approach which, in turn, can allow you to see when qualities in others chime or contrast with your own.

Sometimes, it's all too easy to become lost in the world of endless scrolling, getting pulled into other people's worlds and losing a sense of self along the way. Next time you log on, try tuning in to yourself and notice if you are projecting your own fears, disappointments, failures – as well as your hopes, dreams and talents – onto others. With awareness and patience, it's possible to notice when projection is happening, and noticing can be the first step towards getting to know yourself, in the real world as well as the digital one.

PROJECTION PROTECTION

Eight tips for navigating the psychological complexities of online interaction.

1. Recognise the signs of unhelpful projection in yourself – both projecting onto others (for example, demonising or idealising them, especially based on little evidence or actual contact with the person) and losing touch with yourself. Keep a note of them here as they arise.

....

....

....

....

....

....

....

....

2. Get to know what triggers unhelpful projection in you. Which content or creators (if any) are more likely to make you lose touch with reality?

....

....

....

....

....

....

3. Decide how much you want to curate your feed. Look out for feelings that the digital version of yourself is the real you, or seeing your physical self as not good enough.

....
....
....
....
....
....
....
....

4. Think about when and how you want to receive notifications. It could be you want to stay connected to people but need more control over when you see their content.

....
....
....
....
....
....
....
....
....

5. Choose the way you interact with others. Do you need to respond with a 'like'? Is a comment needed? Might it be helpful to have a cooling-off period before responding? Maybe you'd prefer not to comment at all. Jot down your thoughts.

6. Practise playing with your projections in a positive way. Imagine alternative possibilities and look for more contact to find out which of your projections might be closest to reality.

7. Pause and remember that another person's posts reflect their lived experience, knowledge, fears or hopes – it doesn't make them right or appropriate for you. Are there posts that make you feel you have to imitate or pursue them?

....

....

....

....

....

....

....

....

8. If someone's posts are making you anxious, it might be time to block them. You can do this without them knowing, so you're not going to cause offence. What posts make you feel unsettled?

....

....

....

....

....

....

....

....

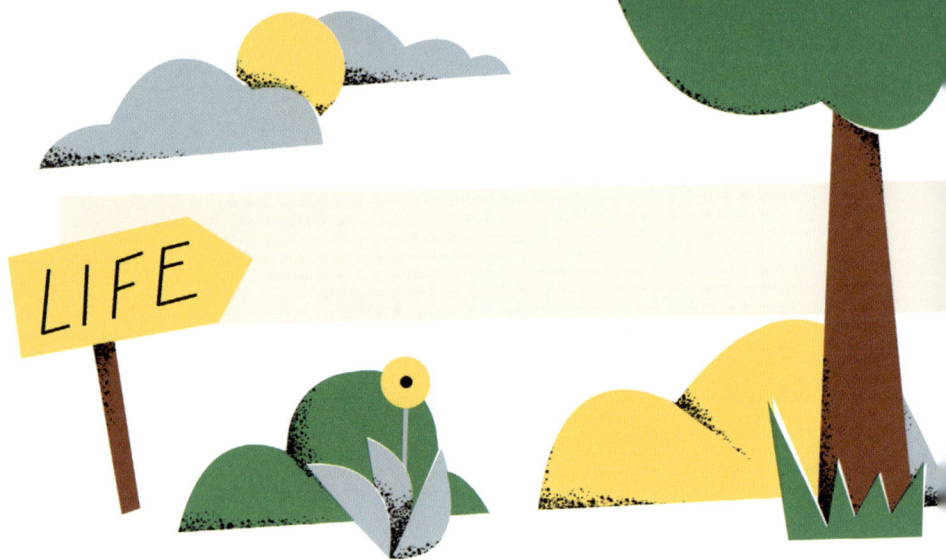

Cogs in motion

Meditation can be a powerful aid when you feel stuck in life. Here we explore ways to get moving again

The gestalt cycle – also known as 'a gestalt' – is a therapeutic model that identifies the seven stages you pass through in any given experience. Used in coaching and education, as well as in personal development, gestalt psychotherapy was founded by German psychoanalysts Laura and Fritz Perls in the 1950s. There is no exact equivalent in English, but the German word 'gestalt' is usually translated as 'whole', 'pattern' or 'form', which reflects the therapy's holistic approach to an individual's experience of the here and now.

What is a gestalt?
A gestalt represents a whole experience that can span varying periods of time. This could mean anything from feeling thirsty and needing a drink of water to situations that require more dramatic action, such as feeling undervalued at work and wanting to find a new job. Clearly, a thirst for water might be a need that's met in one minute, whereas a thirst for a career change might trigger a cycle that spans many years.

Gestalts can occur simultaneously. In fact, the process of a career change will have hundreds – if not thousands – of other gestalts overlapping and interweaving with it. Other gestalts that might occur within a long cycle such as a change of profession could include a need to move house, to resolve a conflict in a relationship or to learn how to play the piano, along with hundreds of other smaller daily gestalts, like the requirement to eat, exercise, spend time with friends, shop for food and complete household tasks.

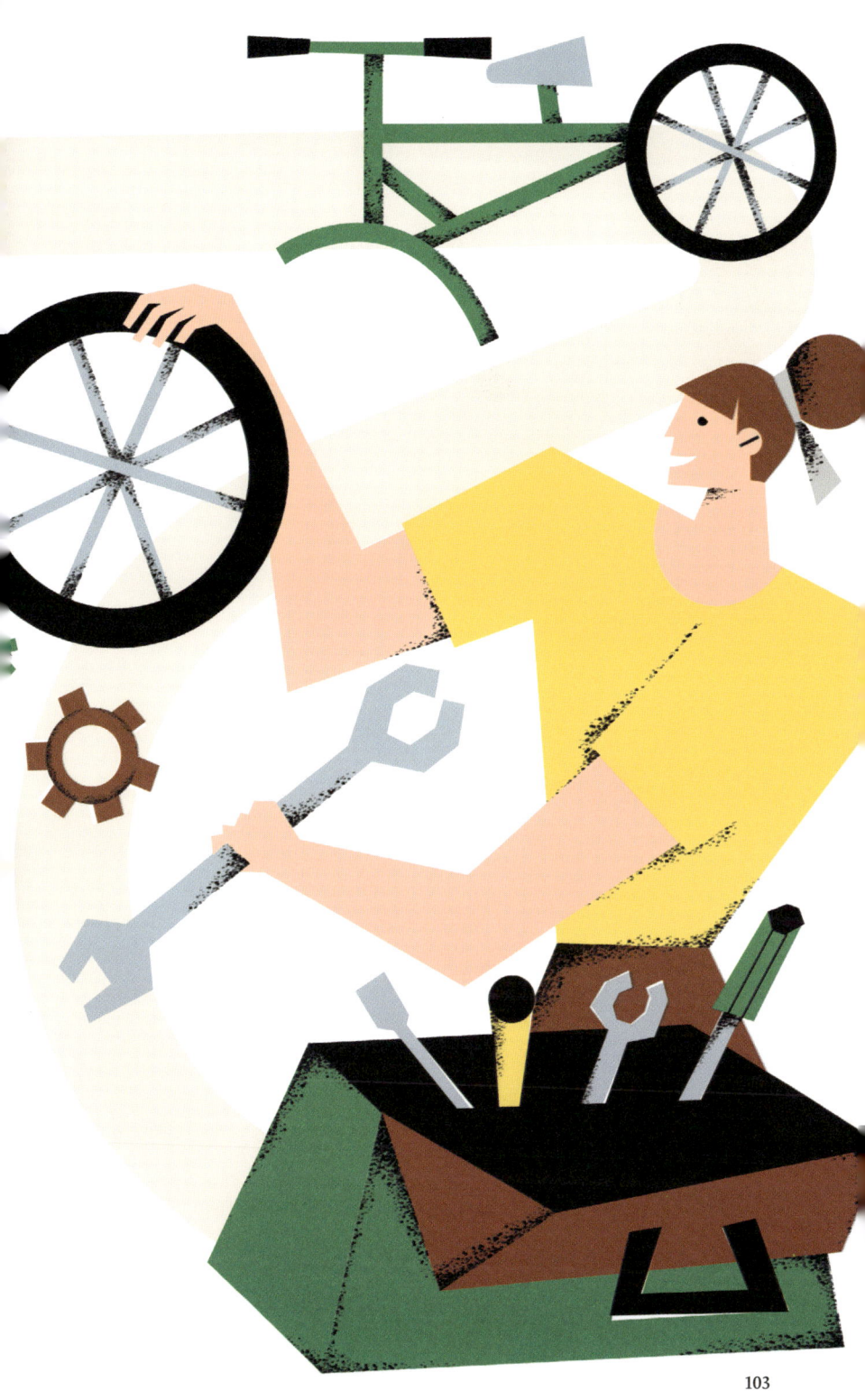

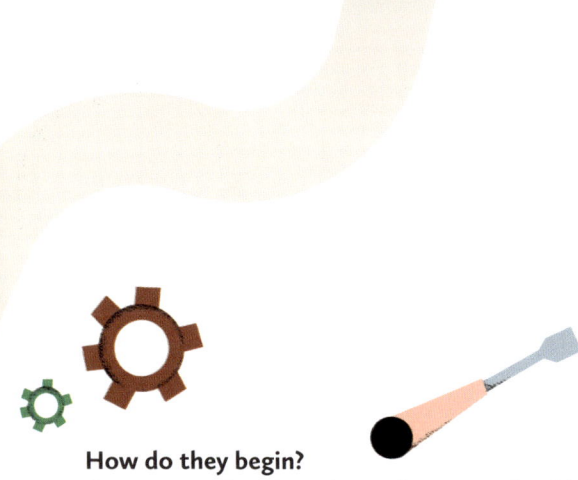

How do they begin?
Common to all cycles is that each starts with a felt sensation. During the course of your life, you experience a multitude of stimuli that you sort through and prioritise automatically. These might be internal sensations, such as tiredness or hunger, emotions that arise, or a sudden idea that occurs to you. Equally, the triggers might be external, such as a knock at the door, the sound of a friend calling you, a job offer or redundancy, or a change in the weather.

Lots of gestalts can happen in the background and you might not bring these experiences fully into your awareness. They might be transient occurrences, things that drift in and out of your day without requiring much thought. Others will feel more significant and might influence the direction of your life, impacting how fulfilled you feel.

Regardless of how big or small they are – or of how much attention you pay to them – each experience will complete a full gestalt, passing through seven distinct phases until the cycle is concluded.

Fertile void
Usually, at the end of a cycle, there's a space before the next sensation occurs. This is called 'the fertile void'. Ideally, in this state, you don't hurry to the next emerging experience, but are willing to experience the pause. When the cycle has been a significant one, this gap might cause unsettled feelings, such as fear or emptiness, and there could be a desire to fill the void with another experience. Or you might bask in the space.

Sometimes, you might find you become stuck at one or more of the stages. Problems could arise that mean a certain phase can't be completed or veers off course. This, in turn, can cause a distortion of the subsequent stages. Tim Carrette, gestalt psychotherapist and course director at Scarborough Counselling & Psychotherapy Training Institute in North Yorkshire, says: 'Everyone can get stuck at any stage or simultaneously at several stages in different cycles. Each episode of "stuckness" is a life lesson. I would say the situation is key here. In gestalt therapy, the situation includes time, place, the people and the relationships involved, and is referred to as "the field". We don't always know when we're stuck, hence the need for relationships with others and therapy.'

Recognising patterns

When you notice your responses to each stage of an experience, you can gain better awareness of your patterns and find solutions to overcome any obstacles or emotions you feel when you're in a rut. A gestalt counsellor or psychotherapist can help you to explore how and why you're experiencing a disturbance in the cycle. It could be that there was a time in the past when it was important that you did disrupt the natural flow of a cycle. Perhaps, for example, you were trying to please a caregiver or you had a different problem to solve that meant you had to make that particular adjustment or sacrifice. In gestalt therapy, these disturbances or interruptions are called creative adjustments. Though useful in the first instance, these adjustments can become habitual and might be less useful, or even detrimental, on subsequent occasions.

Gestalt therapists and coaches believe that it's helpful to notice your disruptions where possible, to act with awareness in the present moment and to take responsibility for the choices you make in your response to a disturbance. 'Recognising that we're stuck involves a raising of awareness,' says Tim. 'Invariably this stuck position, which we call a fixed gestalt, will involve being caught between polarised tensions within the self. The task then is for the therapist to support you to find your authentic truth in relation to the needs of the situation. This may be an individual or a collective or relational need or truth.'

Ever onwards

Once you've learned how to overcome a blockage, it can help you to face future situations with awareness and insight and, hopefully, to find a way forward. 'Once we have enough energy and the time is right, we can take action,' says Tim. 'Appropriate action in the right place at the right time creates contact. Contact then leads to either satisfaction or another lesson, and the cycle repeats.' Gestalts are, like all cycles, a continuous process. The aim is to learn how to keep rolling.

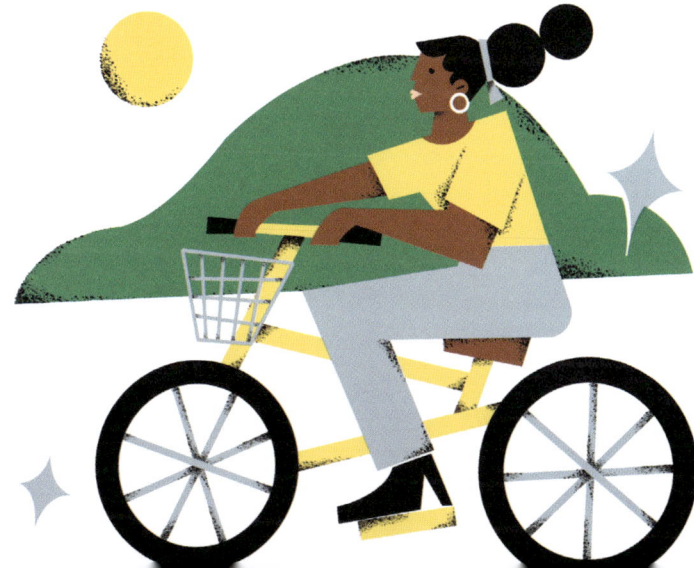

THE SEVEN STAGES OF A GESTALT

1. Sensation
This is when you experience a stimulus from the environment or from within. A sense of dissatisfaction could arise. You might hear the sound of an alarm clock, for example, or get a bodily signal, such as experiencing a dry mouth.

2. Recognition or awareness
You become aware of the sensation, attempting to recognise it and name it. Perhaps you feel listless or thirsty. Sensations can be read differently – a tight chest to one person might be interpreted as anxiety but for another it might be seen as the possible start of a cold or virus.

3. Mobilisation of energy
This is where you respond to the stimuli, try to make sense of it and consider what to do about it. You prepare to act – you make a simple decision to get a drink, for example, or a complex one to retrain in a new field.

4. Action
This is where you make a movement towards your goal. You might experiment with different routes of action until you find the most satisfactory one for you. Your plan is then put into action – you walk into the kitchen and make a drink or set about updating your CV.

5. Contact
At this stage, you're fully engaged with whatever you've chosen to do and you focus all of your senses on the experience. You take a sip of that drink and are fully in that moment, savouring the taste, or are immersed in the recruitment process.

6. Satisfaction
If your need has been met with full contact, you'll feel a sense of completion and satisfaction at this stage (even if the interaction was a challenging one, such as an expression of frustration in the form of tears). Regardless, a sense of relief will be experienced, such as the enjoyment of your thirst being quenched or pride in your new role.

7. Withdrawal
This is the final stage and where you withdraw your attention from your experience and naturally lose interest. The gestalt is complete. You have let go of the experience now that you're satisfied.

THE SEVEN CAUSES OF GETTING STUCK

1. Desensitisation
Your natural ability to sense and feel the world is numbed.

2. Deflection
You divert energy from its natural path to an alternative one.

3. Introjection
You absorb or 'swallow' whole a rule or message – something from the past that has been accepted without discrimination.

4. Projection
You disown an aspect of yourself and place it on another person, animal or object.

5. Retroflection
When energy which would usually be directed outwards is turned inwards – for example, stopping yourself from speaking out and biting your lip instead.

6. Egotism
The process of self-monitoring, such as noticing how you're performing and fixating on that, instead of moving forward in the cycle.

7. Confluence
You merge with the environment, so a sense of individuality is lost, and it becomes difficult to separate your own experience from someone else's.

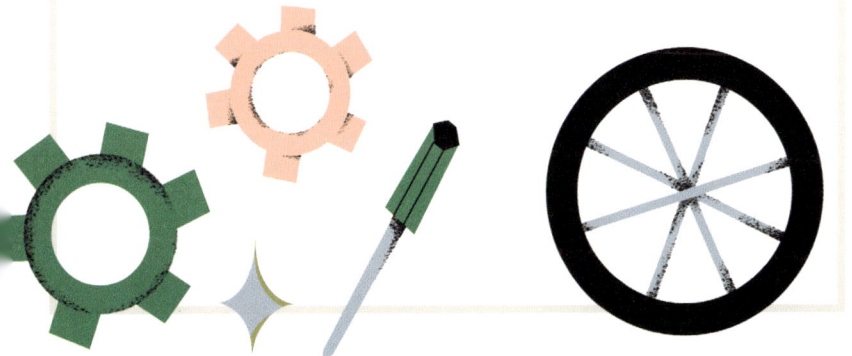

HOW TO GET A CYCLE MOVING AGAIN

Try the following courses of action:

Be aware
Start by trying to cultivate awareness of your everyday gestalts (experiences). Meditation can be a powerful tool for this. Similar to using mindfulness techniques, try to begin to notice and become conscious of what's happening in your world.

Share with others
The third stage of the cycle is mobilisation of energy. If you get stuck here, this is where your relationality or interrelatedness comes in. By sharing your dilemma with others, you can gather energy. Sometimes, this takes the form of encouragement, while on other occasions it will be a challenge. Both are supportive in generating impetus.

Reflect on your 'shoulds'
Often, these stuck places are complex and involve dealing with rules and expectations from the past. Use the space here to list all the 'shoulds' you encounter in daily life or during a given experience. Examples of this might be feeling obliged to attend a work party even though you don't want to, or believing that wasting food is wrong, so you should finish your dinner regardless of whether you're full.

....

....

....

....

....

....

....

....

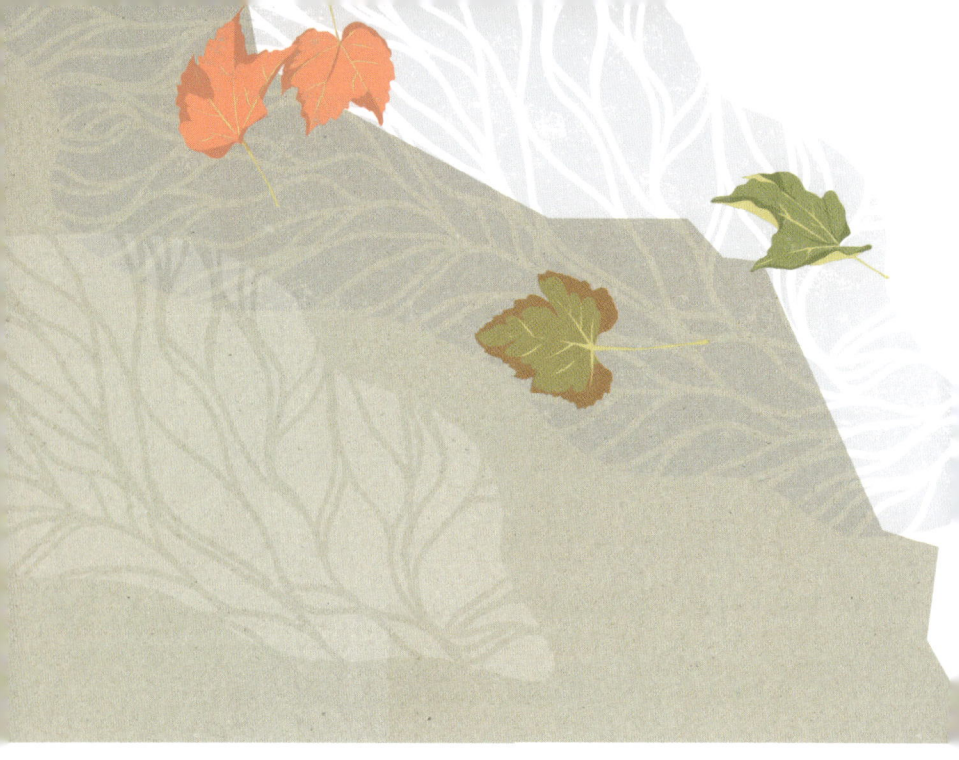

Reawaken the senses

Modern life is awash with millions of messages, many of which are screened out by the brain to prevent people becoming overwhelmed and unable to function. Sometimes, however, this necessary process can also mean losing touch with experiences that bring joy

If you watch a toddler for a few minutes, you'll probably notice that they're constantly looking, listening, smelling, tasting and touching. This learning behaviour continues during the first decade of a child's life as they use their senses to feed their curiosity about the world around them – and turn into question-asking machines in the process.

As they enter adolescence, however, they begin to see and learn about the world through their emotions more than their senses. In adulthood, sensory learning becomes further narrowed as one sense comes to dominate, pushing the others into the background. Of all the sensory learning styles, it is generally visual (seeing), auditory (listening) or kinaesthetic (physical feeling and awareness) that take centre stage.

Stimulation overload

This reduction in awareness is exacerbated, somewhat counter-intuitively, by sensory overload, which is a by-product of modern lifestyles. Every day, a huge number of words assail the eyes and the ears through TV, print, the internet, radio, phone messages, emails and social media. Quoted in *The New York Times*, professor of technology management Roger Bohn said: 'Print media has declined consistently, but if you add up the amount of time people spend surfing the web, they are actually reading more than ever.'

For those living in urban areas – estimated to be 56.2 per cent of the world's population in 2020, according to information from the United Nations' Population Division – there's also the added stimuli of noise and air pollution. Those car horns, police sirens, diesel fumes, billboards and piped music take their toll. This prompts the brain to begin filtering out irrelevant stimuli – a process called sensory gating – in order to ease the stress and avoid a situation where the person becomes overwhelmed.

Unfortunately, the combined impact of both age- and sensory-related gating can mean a significant reduction in some of life's greatest sensory pleasures. Luckily, however, with vigilance and regular practice of focused exercises, it's possible to reawaken the senses one by one and then bring them back together again for a full sensory experience.

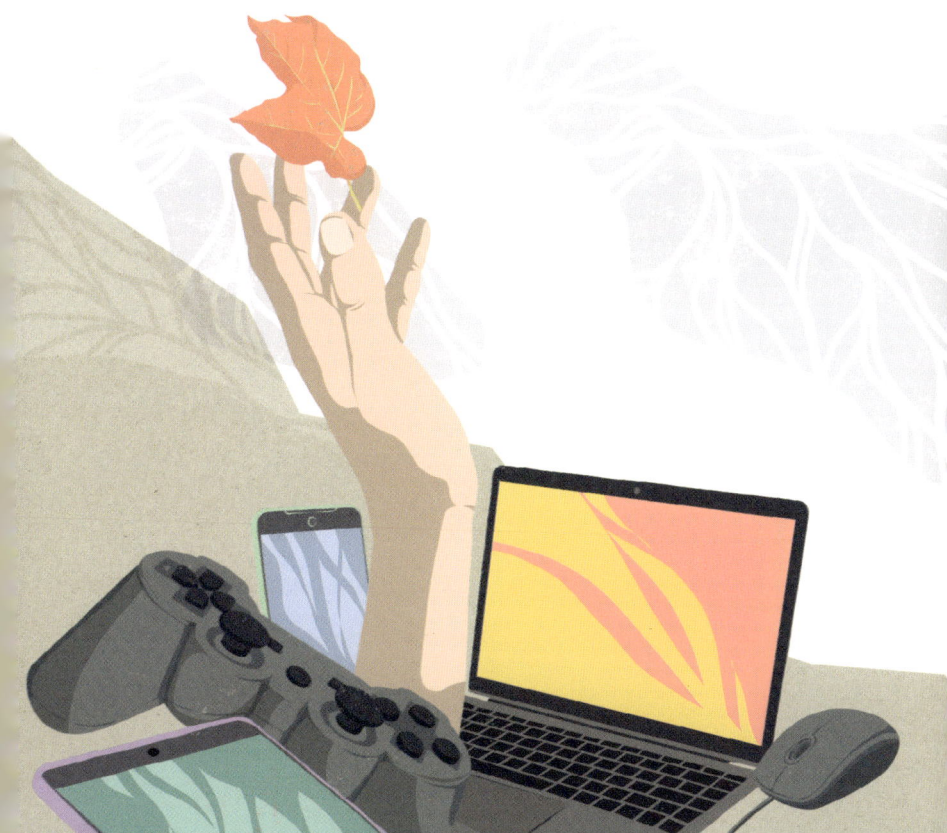

RETUNE INTO THE WORLD AROUND YOU

Sight
Sight is the strongest sense, accounting for about 80 per cent of all sensory input. Yet there are times when visual autopilot kicks in. This is when what is known as the brain's default mode network is active. If you've ever driven home from work or the shops and struggled to recall what happened en route, the chances are your brain was on visual autopilot. The same thing might happen if you were out walking in the forest and your brain was so preoccupied with thoughts of to-do lists or family worries that it missed the beautiful surroundings and the benefits of being in nature.

Sight can also be adversely affected by technology. In 2019, a study at the University of Pittsburgh Medical Center found that too much screen time can cause short-sightedness and reduce focus flexibility. It can also result in dry eyes as people tend to blink less often when using screens. To reduce eye fatigue, they suggested using the 20-20-20 rule, which involves taking a screen break every 20 minutes, where for 20 seconds you look into the distance to a point at least 20 metres away. In 2021, the *Journal of the American Medical Association* published results from a large longitudinal study of schoolchildren in China. Results showed that less time spent outside and increased screen time indoors because of Covid-19 restrictions had almost doubled the incidence of myopia.

Try this exercise...
To borrow a photographic term, you can change your visual focal length from close-up to long distance to rest your eyes. Spend a minute standing in one spot and look out into the distance. What can you see? Hold that long-distance focus and, without moving your eyes, check your peripheral vision, which can be as wide as 170°. What can you see? Notice all the detail in the wide field of view. This is known as being in visual expanded awareness.

Visual awareness of beauty in the environment can also create a sense of awe and a feeling of being part of something grander, which according to some studies – including the 2016 paper, *Standing in Awe: The Effects of Awe on Body Perception and the Relation with Absorption*, by Michiel van Elk et al – can help to decrease levels of depression, anxiety, loneliness and pain, while increasing wellbeing.

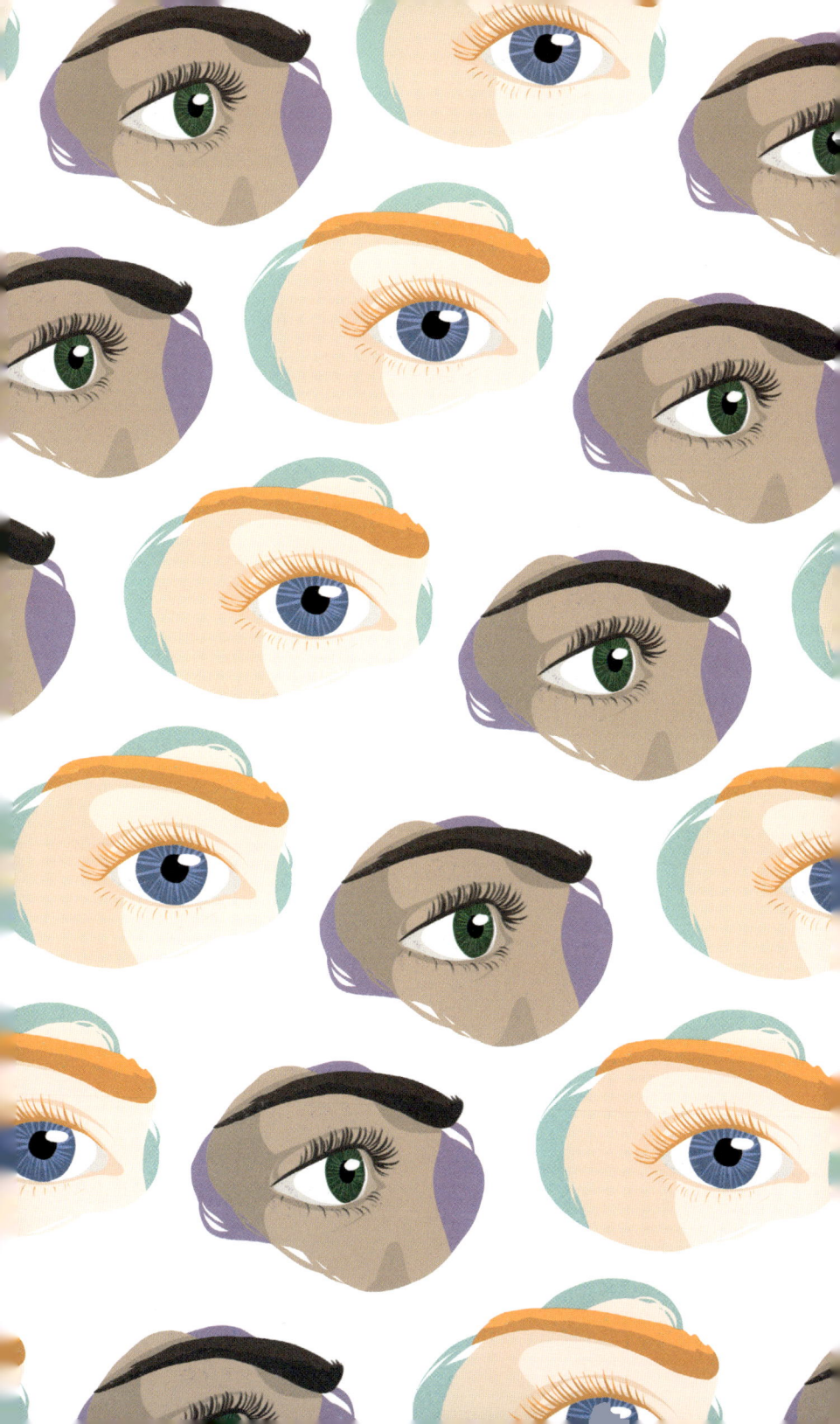

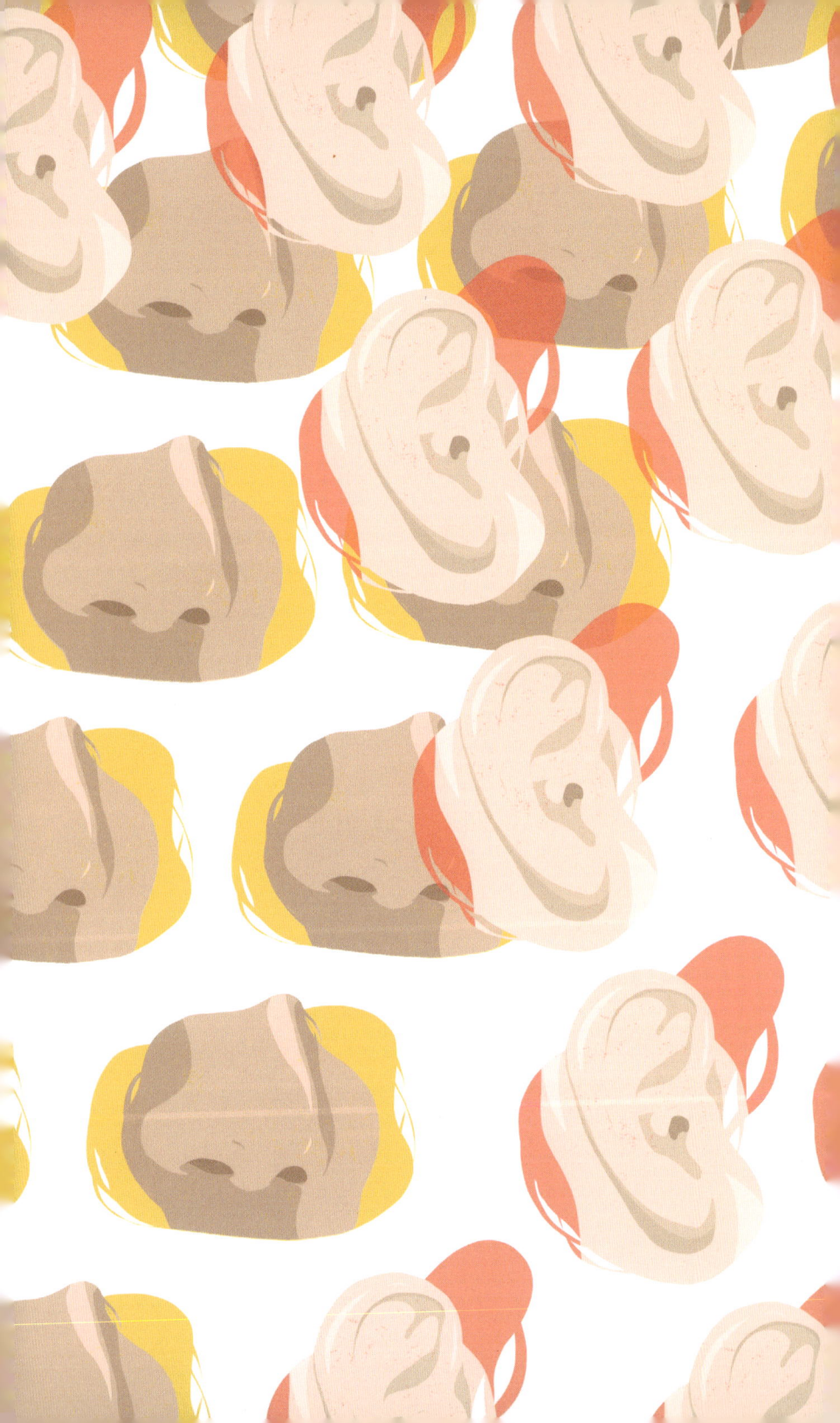

Smell
The Harvard Brain Science Initiative studied how scent, emotion and memory were intertwined. Smell receptors send messages, via the limbic system, to the amygdala and hippocampus, where emotions and memories are formed. A certain aroma, for example, can transport a person straight back to a childhood holiday or bring to mind days out with a loved one.

However, mindfulness organisations such as Headspace say that, over time, the instinctive breathing patterns people are born with have been compromised by environmental factors that have encouraged shallow rather than deep breathing. Culprits include air pollution, loud noise and extremes in temperature, both hot and cold. In turn, this has had an effect on cognitive function and the ability to store memories.

Try this exercise...
Inhaling deeply through the nose enhances the sense of smell and stimulates various systems in the brain. Try using box breathing. Ideally do this outside when you are sitting somewhere comfortable. Inhale through your nose for a count of four, noticing what you can smell. Hold the breath for another four seconds, breathe out through your mouth for four seconds and hold for another four. Do this four times to see how many things you can smell. Remember, too, that the smells can be anything – they're not limited to freshly cut grass, fragrant roses or a waft of coffee from a local cafe. You might notice Tarmac or petrichor, for example.

Sound
City dwellers are often so used to traffic noise that it no longer registers, but in zoning out what might be unwelcome sounds, is there also a danger that more uplifting ones might be masked? What if morning birdsong, for example, is missed when zoning out becomes the norm? The Acoustical Society of America studied this and found that listening to sounds fell into two areas:

- Conscious listening, such as trying hard to note everything during a hearing test.
- Selective hearing (known as auditory selective attention), where people tune out certain sounds.

Try this exercise...
To tune into your hearing, temporarily shut down your strongest sense, which for most people will be sight, and listen for sounds. There could be birds chirping, dogs barking or leaves rustling. You might also hear mechanical noises, maybe the drone of an aircraft or the trundle of a train. Now focus solely on a sound you find restful in all the auditory chaos, be that birds or trains, and note as many qualities about it as you can – the pitch, the volume, the intensity.

Taste
How often do you sit down and focus your full attention on what you're eating? It can be difficult when there's work to be done or family to be looked after. Toast might be eaten while leaving the house and lunch grabbed quickly between work or home tasks.

Research conducted in 2014 by healthcare and insurance group BUPA found that almost a third of UK office workers regularly ate lunch while sitting at their desks, while *The New York Times* reported that 62 per cent of professionals in the US did the same, a habit known as desktop dining. This can result in what nutritionists call unconscious eating or eating without thinking.

Try this exercise...
The brain's perception of how an item of food or a drink is going to taste is intrinsically tied to how it smells (how it looks can also have an effect). Tastebuds register salty, sweet, sour, bitter and umami, which trigger different areas on the tongue.

One way to isolate taste from smell is to hold your nose while you have food in your mouth and notice which part of the tongue is triggered. Then breathe in through your nose and notice all the flavours. If you want to really test yourself, enlist the help of a friend, and ask them to pass you different foods to eat while you keep your eyes closed, hold your nose, then let go and breathe in.

Touch
The skin, the body's biggest organ, sends messages to the brain about the outside environment, enabling it to register temperature, texture or the brush of a breeze. And with touch, comes physical feeling. To touch something is to come into contact with it. To feel it, is to be aware you are touching it and how it feels. It's easy to become blasé or even numb to the experience of touch and feeling.

Oxytocin, sometimes referred to as the hug hormone, is released with touch. The recent health emergency, which saw people around the world discouraged from shaking hands, putting a comforting arm around a friend or hugging loved ones, could mean that many are lacking in oxytocin.

Try this exercise...
If it's safe to do so, touch and hug those you love. Pet owners can also happily get lots of oxytocin by stroking their animals. If you don't have a pet, visit a city farm or ask a friend if it's okay to borrow theirs for a small squeeze.

Grounding, meanwhile, is one way to notice what you feel. Go walking barefoot on sand, grass, in water or all three. Feel the warm sun on your skin, grainy sand or blades of grass underfoot, cool water around your ankles and the breeze through your hair. You might notice feeling calmer with a release of happy hormones.

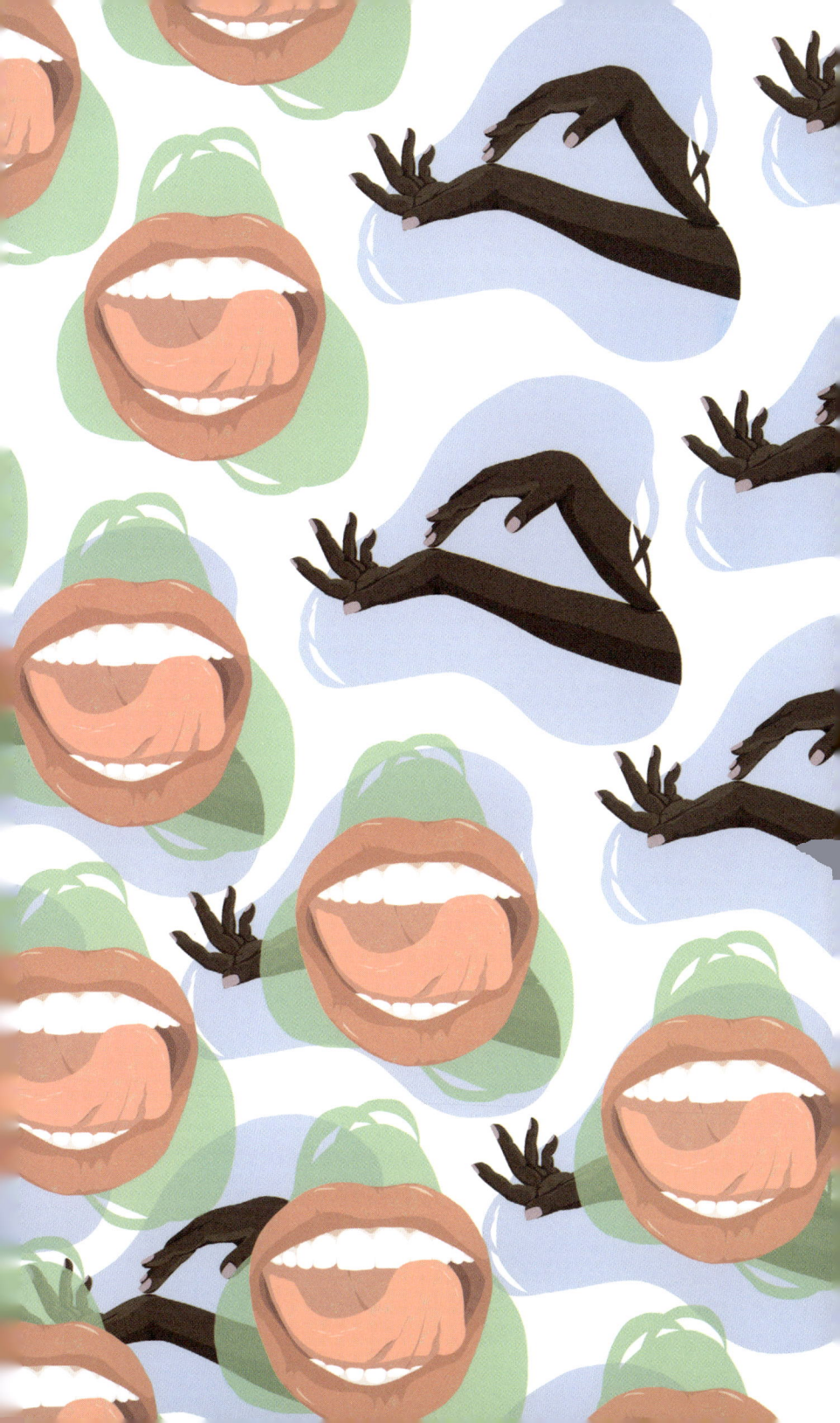

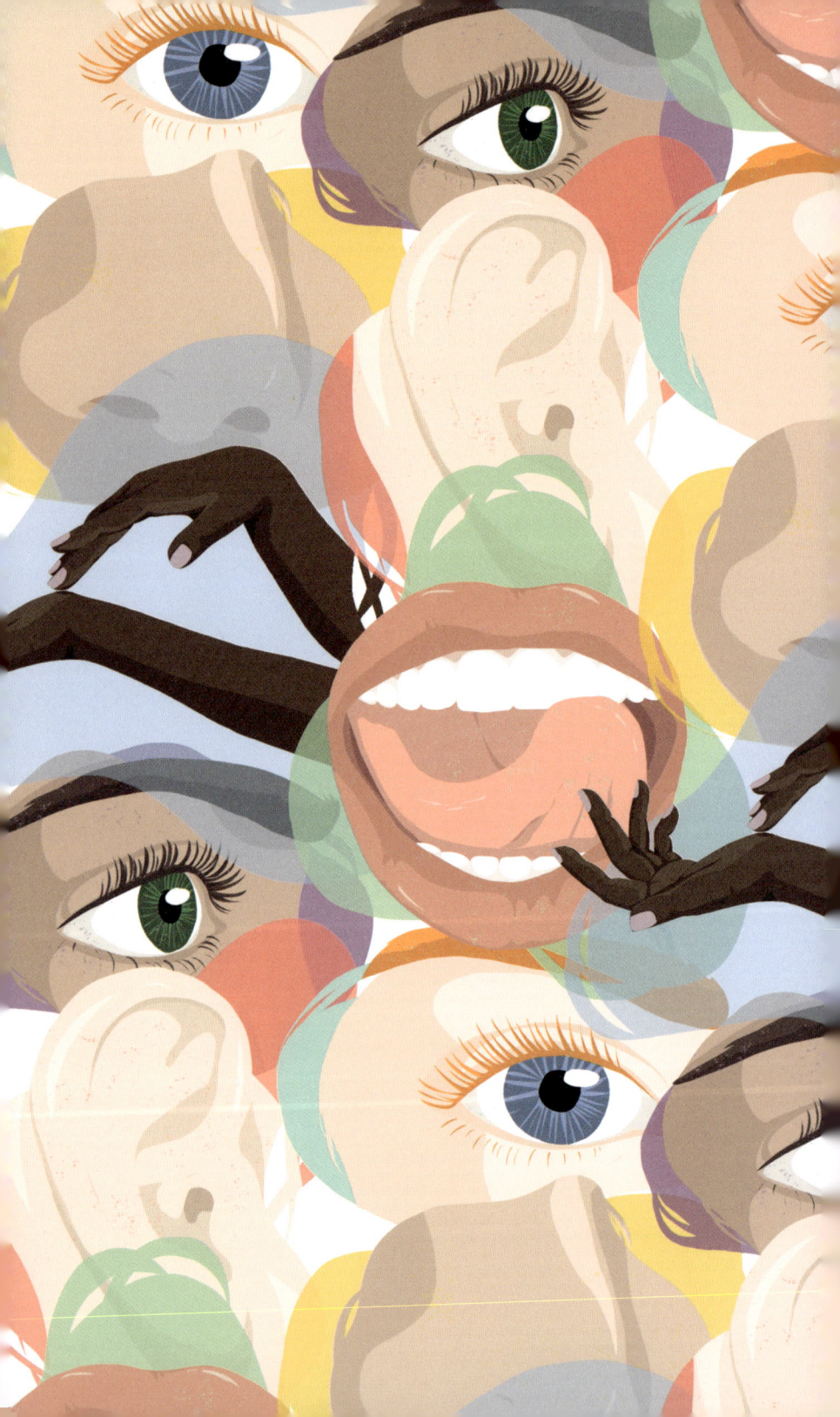

60-SECOND SENSORY RESET

Sometimes you might notice your senses are fading, be that because of work or family pressure, ongoing distractions or tuning out unpleasant experiences. If this happens, try this wake-up-your-senses mindful exercise to get you into the moment. It can be done anywhere, any time when feeling overwhelmed.

Sight
Step outside, where there's a view into the distance. Keeping your eyes focused ahead, stretch your arms out on both sides of your body. Wiggle your fingers. You should be able to see your fingers with your peripheral vision.

Smell
Inhale deeply through your nose for a count of four seconds, and exhale for four. Pause and notice what you can smell.

Hearing
Close your eyes. Tune into and listen to the sounds around you. What can you hear?

Taste
Grab some food or drink. Hold your nose, pop the food into your mouth. Chew a little and let go of your nose. What do you taste?

Touch
Do a quick body scan. This can be done anywhere. From head to toe, notice what you can feel on your skin: cool, hot, pressure. Can you feel a breeze on your face? Are your hands hot or cold? Which part of the body is touching another object, like a chair or clothing?

'The five senses are the ministers of the soul'

Leonardo da Vinci

Slowly but surely

It's important to take time to relax at the end of a busy day, and meditation can help to restore mental and physical energy. But what can you do if trying to wind down is winding you up?

Relaxation is an important element of a healthy lifestyle, so why do some of us find it so hard to enter a truly restful and restorative state? Imagine a car pootling along at 20 miles an hour. It will take 12 metres to come to a stop, but the braking distance of a car driving at 70 miles per hour is a whopping 96 metres. Similarly the faster paced and more hectic a person's lifestyle is, the longer it will take them to slow down. Most people cannot slip easily from full speed to zen, so simply scheduling a meditation at the end of a busy day is probably not going to cut it.

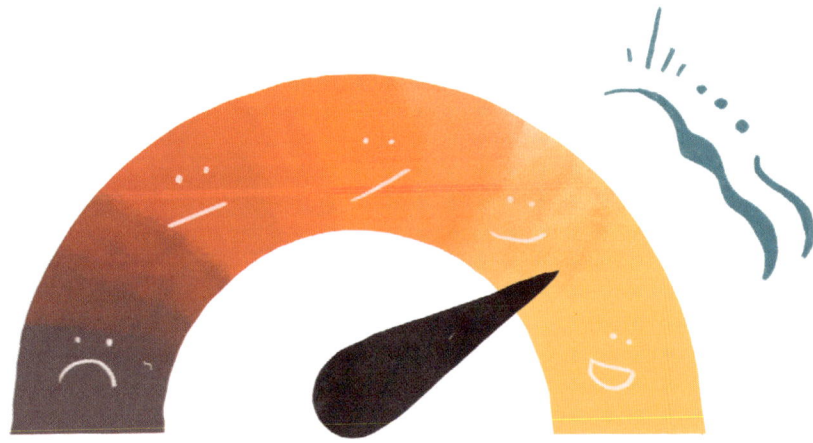

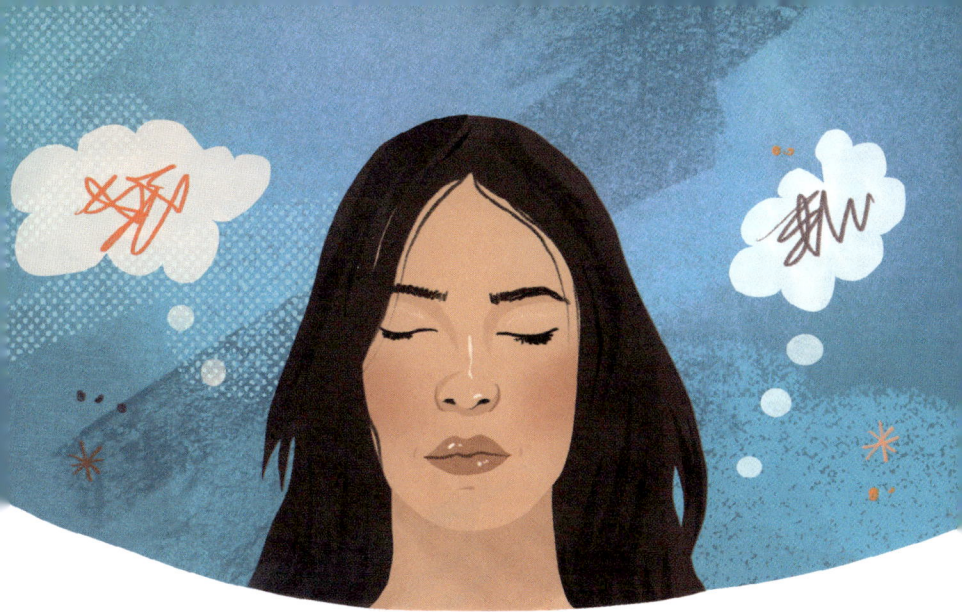

Drawing a line

The pressure to be productive is potent. With work and the world at large so readily accessible through a tiny screen on our phones, it can be difficult to know when and how to withdraw. Wired from an on-the-go lifestyle, shutting down a busy mind for a while can sometimes feel impossible. This is partly because during the day our bodies produce chemical messengers, known as neurotransmitters, in response to activities that stimulate the mind or body. Some of them, such as adrenaline, help us stay alert and fuel our productivity. But they're not compatible with a state of calm and it can take up to an hour for their effects to subside. When this happens, and the signs indicate that it's a struggle to get into the relaxation zone, it can be useful to make time for the winding-down process. Getting into a routine that signals to the mind and body that it's time to take it easy can make this easier.

Towards the end of your day, for example, schedule tasks that are less physically or mentally stimulating. If you have a sedentary job, you might find you need to use up some energy before you can unwind in which case you could try to increase your physical activity throughout the day by making small changes to your routine. If you're based at home and don't get a chance to decompress on your commute, it might help to do some exercise after you finish for the day. Try taking a walk, going for a run or doing an exercise class – there are many online options if you can't make it in person. This helps to create a line between active and relaxation time. The brain also responds well to sensory signals so listening to music, burning incense, lighting a candle or talking to a friend can all form part of your calming process.

WHAT'S STANDING IN YOUR WAY?

Of course, there are many obstacles that might make it difficult to wind down. Here are a few:

'I don't have time'
Relaxation doesn't have to be time-consuming. It can be as simple and quick as taking a few calming breaths into the diaphragm at regular intervals throughout the day, choosing to step away from a stressful situation for a bit or taking a moment or two to gaze out of the window. Recognise the natural pauses in your day and allow yourself to enjoy them without feeling the need to fill them with productivity. When you plan your schedule, make sure that you create buffer zones to allow for taking stock before embarking on the next set of tasks.

'I can't relax until everything is done'
Don't fall into the trap of waiting until your to-do list is complete, as for most people, it never is. We're not designed to work flat out all day. Instead, energy levels go through a cycle of peaks and troughs. Notice when your body is urging you to rest (usually every one-and-a-half to two hours) and when you're finding it difficult to concentrate or be productive. If you take heed of these prompts, you might find your energy levels are more sustainable. And it's often in the quiet, still moments that inspiration pops up.

'I'm too wired'
The idea of winding down at the end of the day is a misnomer. It implies it's acceptable to be wound up for the duration of the day. If you are too stimulated to rest in the evening and a decompression routine is not enough then it might help to look at levelling out stress levels throughout the day by changing your routines.

'I don't like sitting still'
You can be calm without being totally stationary. Gentle, restorative exercise like qigong, tai chi, Pilates, body balance, yoga, golf, walking, swimming and dancing will all help to elicit the relaxation response. Work out what helps you to loosen up and do more of it.

'My mind races'
You set aside time to unwind and as soon as you sit down, your head is filled with thoughts of everything that needs doing. If this happens to you, it might be time to do a little negotiating with the taskmaster in your brain. Reassure your busy mind that those things will get done. It might help to write your to-do list for the next day or make a plan as part of your winding-down process.

'I feel guilty'
Many people find themselves conflating busyness with self-worth. But you can't keep running on an empty fuel tank. Acknowledge the thoughts and feelings that come up when trying to take a break. They might offer insight into deeply held beliefs that need updating.

'Relaxation makes me stressed'
Knowing that we should relax can often lead us to put pressure on ourselves. Any internal dialogue that includes vocabulary like 'should', 'ought to', 'must' and 'have to' are likely to cause stress and make peacefulness feel even more unattainable. Tranquillity will not look the same for everyone. Be open to trying new ways to kick back while also thinking about things that have brought calm in the past.

The important thing is to try not to make unwinding another item to be ticked off a never-ending to-do list. If possible, remember that relaxation isn't something to do, rather it's something to feel.

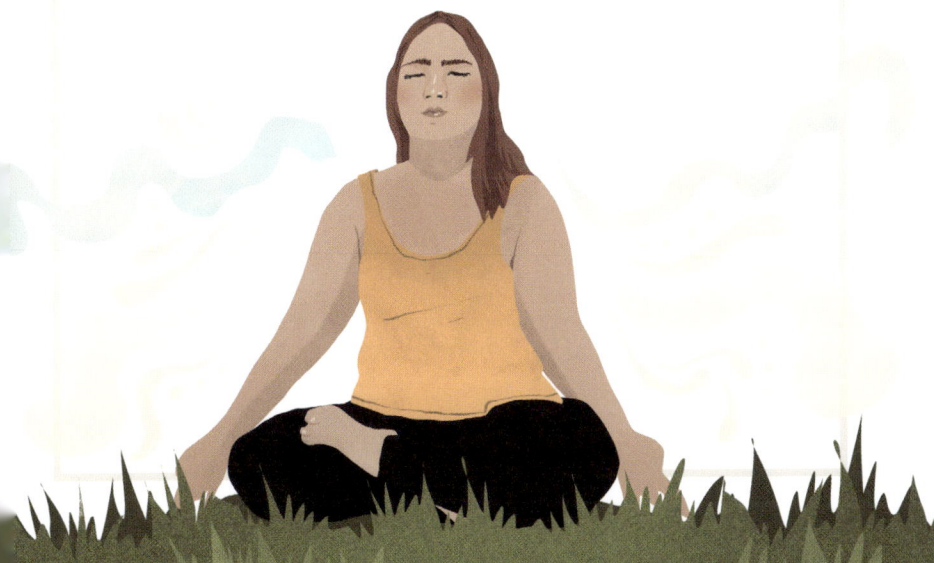

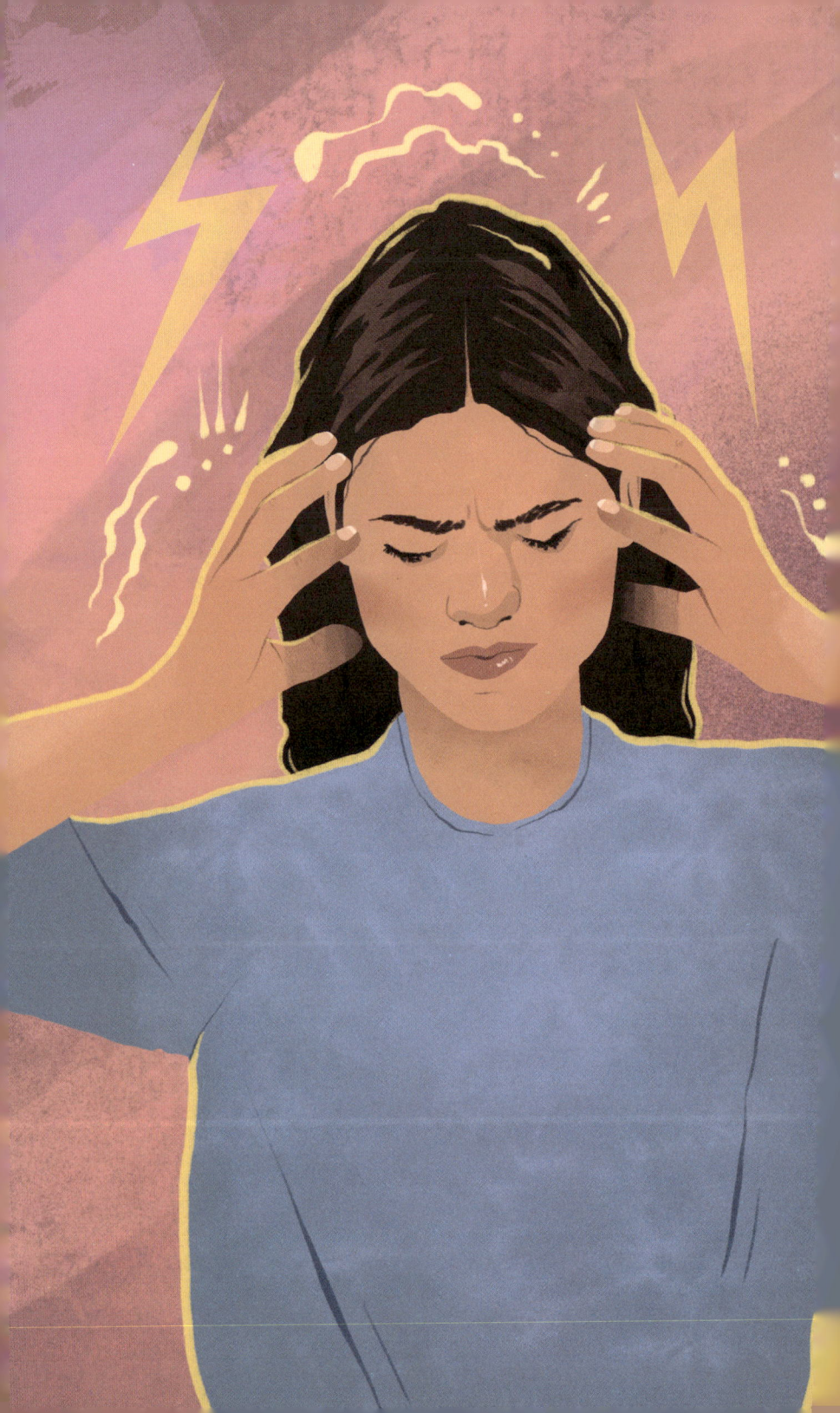

CAN'T GET INTO THE ZONE?

Signs you might be struggling to get into relaxation mode:

- Multitasking even during leisure time, such as scrolling through social media while watching TV.

- Finding it hard to switch off from work and other responsibilities.

- Doing nothing prompts anxiety or guilt.

- Experiencing difficulty getting to sleep even when exhaustion has set in.

- Feeling tired even after seven or eight hours' sleep.

- Engaging in peaceful activities fails to stop fidgeting or boredom.

- Insisting all tasks and chores are done before sitting down.

- Exhausting all energy reserves before allowing a period of inactivity.

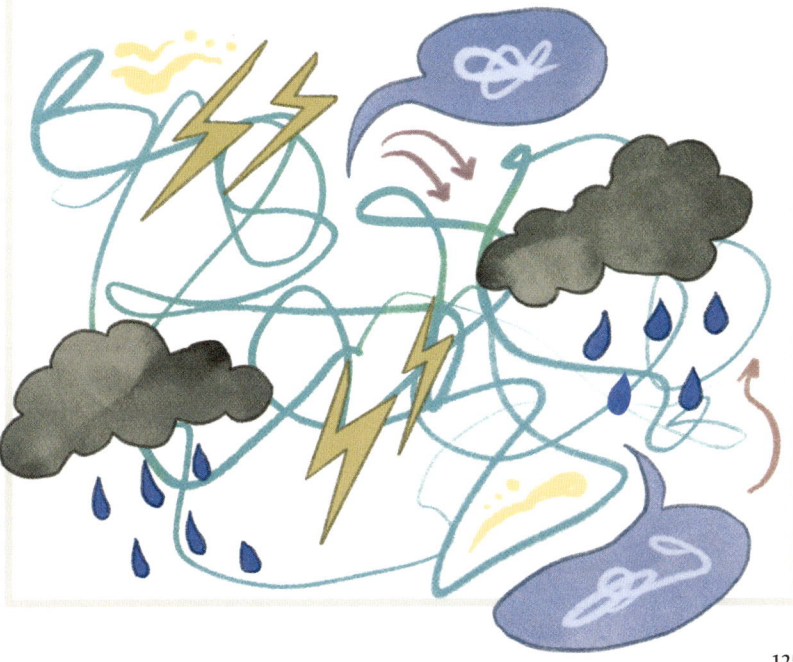

INACTION PLAN

Ways to deepen relaxation:

- Practise breathing into your belly and sighing out your breath.

- Take regular media breaks, particularly during the first hour of the day and the last hour before you go to bed.

- Visit a peaceful place in your mind, maybe somewhere you've been on holiday that you loved.

- Get out and enjoy nature. A walk in a local park can work magic.

- Do things you enjoy, whether it's reading a book or magazine, taking a nap or lazing in a scented bath.

- Try a restorative exercise such as yoga or a meditation class.

- Explore your creativity without worrying about the end result. Knit, paint or sew for the fun of it.

- Listen to music without feeling the need to be doing something else at the same time.

- Use the spotlight of your attention to scan your body, noticing the sensations you find there.

- Concentrate on a low-stakes task like a jigsaw, crossword or colouring.

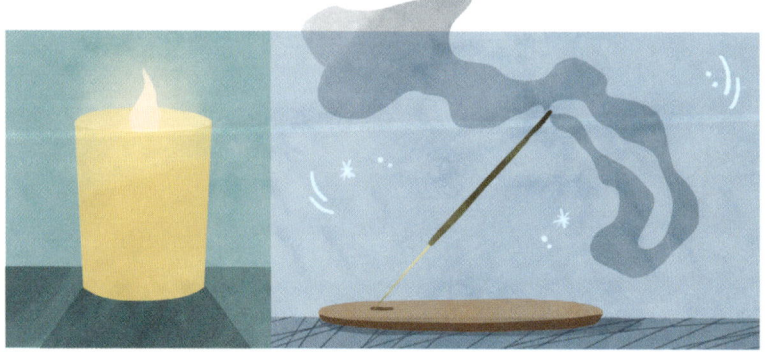

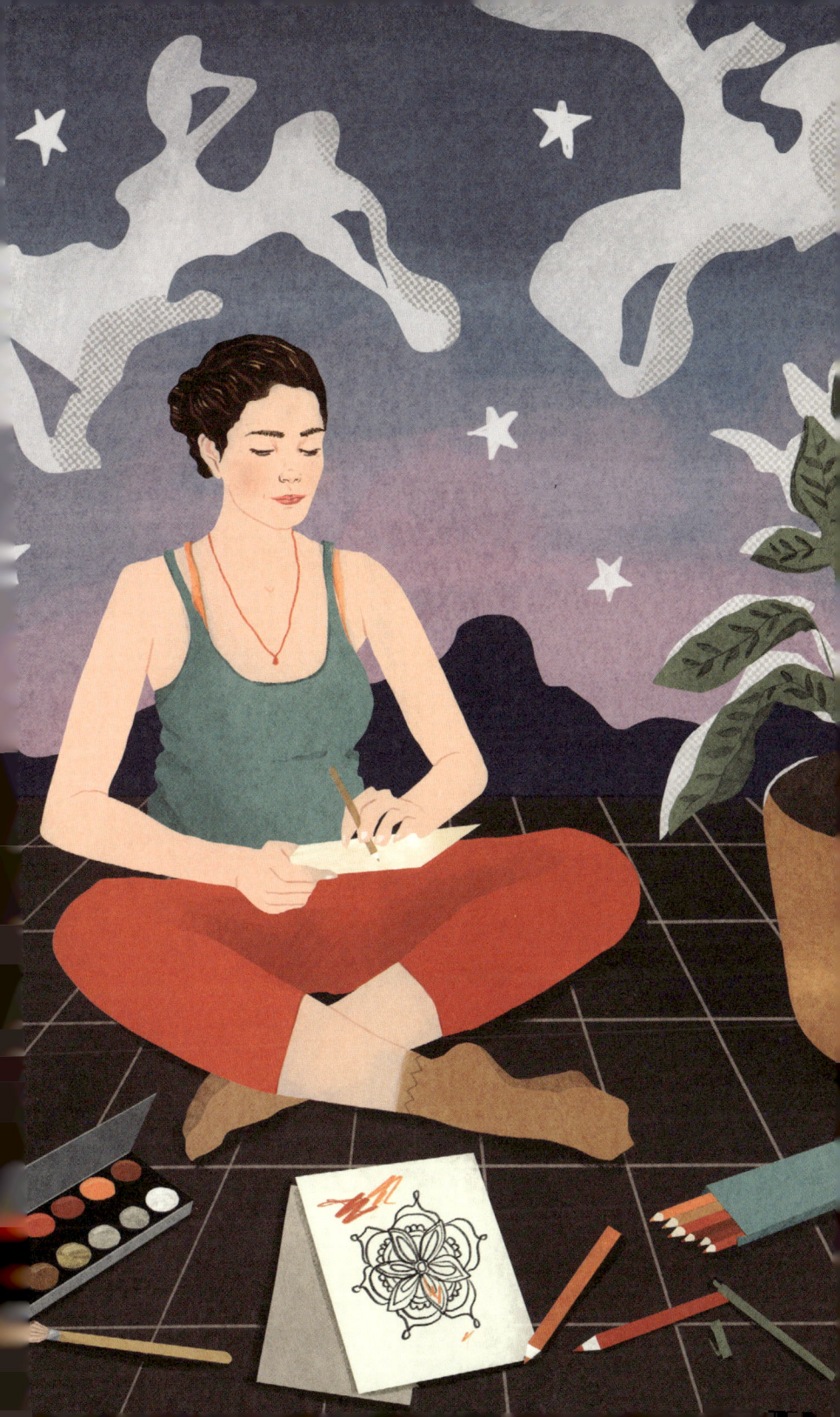

Breathe

BREATHE is a trademark of Guild of Master Craftsman Publications Ltd

First published 2023 by
Ammonite Press
an imprint of Guild of Master Craftsman Publications Ltd
Castle Place, 166 High Street, Lewes, East Sussex BN7 1XU, United Kingdom

www.ammonitepress.com
www.breathemagazine.com

Copyright in the Work © GMC Publications Ltd, 2023

Compiled by Susie Duff
Editorial: Catherine Kielthy, Jane Roe, Josie Fletcher
Words credits: Jade Beecroft, Jillian Bell, Kerry Dolan, Samhita Foria, Yvonne Gavan, Heather Grant,
Leah Larwood, Kate Orson, Jane Pelusey, Emma Powell, Angharad Rudkin

Illustrations: Magda Azab, Louise Billyard, Tonwen Jones, Irina Perju, Katie Smith,
Silvia Stecher, Maggie Stephenson, Michelle Urra
Cover illustration: Kate Styling

ISBN 978 1 78145 481 7

All rights reserved.

No part of this publication may be reproduced, stored in a retrieval system, or transmitted in any form or by any means (including electronic, mechanical, photocopying, recording, or otherwise) without prior written permission from the publisher.

The publishers can accept no legal responsibility for any consequences arising from the application of information, advice or instructions given in this publication.

A catalogue record for this book is available from the British Library.

Breathe Magazine
Publisher: Jonathan Grogan

Colour reproduction by GMC Reprographics
Printed and bound in China

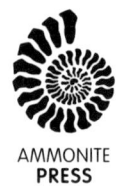

AMMONITE
PRESS